Essentials in Ophthalmology

Series Editor:

Arun D. Singh
Cleveland Clinic Foundation
Cole Eye Institute
Cleveland, OH, USA

Essentials in Ophthalmology aims to promote the rapid and efficient transfer of medical research into clinical practice. It is published in four volumes per year. Covering new developments and innovations in all fields of clinical ophthalmology, it provides the clinician with a review and summary of recent research and its implications for clinical practice. Each volume is focused on a clinically relevant topic and explains how research results impact diagnostics, treatment options and procedures as well as patient management.

The reader-friendly volumes are highly structured with core messages, summaries, tables, diagrams and illustrations and are written by internationally well-known experts in the field. A volume editor supervises the authors in his/her field of expertise in order to ensure that each volume provides cutting-edge information most relevant and useful for clinical ophthalmologists. Contributions to the series are peer reviewed by an editorial board.

More information about this series at http://www.springer.com/series/5332

Asim V. Farooq • James J. Reidy
Editors

Blepharitis

A Comprehensive Clinical Guide

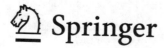 Springer

Editors
Asim V. Farooq
Department of Ophthalmology
& Visual Science
University of Chicago Medical Center
Chicago, IL
USA

James J. Reidy
Department of Ophthalmology
& Visual Science
University of Chicago Medical Center
Chicago, IL
USA

ISSN 1612-3212   ISSN 2196-890X   (electronic)
Essentials in Ophthalmology
ISBN 978-3-030-65042-1   ISBN 978-3-030-65040-7   (eBook)
https://doi.org/10.1007/978-3-030-65040-7

This Springer imprint is published by the registered company Springer Nature Switzerland AG
The registered company address is: Gewerbestrasse 11, 6330 Cham, Switzerland

To our mentors, David J. Apple, MD, Herbert E. Kaufman, MD, and Joel Sugar, MD.

Preface

Blepharitis is one of the most commonly encountered diagnoses in the clinical practice of ophthalmology. However, the term blepharitis is nonspecific and represents many different conditions that can cause a common set of signs and symptoms. Over the past decade, an international consensus regarding classification, diagnosis, and management of blepharitis has been established by a panel of experts from around the world. This text, targeted for eye care professionals, will provide a concise, up-to-date review of the classification, diagnosis, and treatment of blepharitis. It is not meant to be an exhaustive reference, but rather a useful clinic primer.

While there is much about the varied aspects of blepharitis that remains unknown, advances in diagnostic technology, microbiology, genomics, proteomics, and metabolomics will continue to enhance our understanding of these disease processes and ultimately lead to more effective treatment strategies for our patients.

Chicago, IL, USA

Asim V. Farooq, MD
James J. Reidy, MD, FACS

Acknowledgments

The editors wish to gratefully acknowledge the invaluable assistance of Ms. Tracy Marton.

Contents

Contributors

Charles S. Bouchard, MD, MA Loyola University Medical Center, Department of Ophthalmology, Maywood, IL, USA

Asim V. Farooq, MD University of Chicago, Chicago, IL, USA

Farida E. Hakim University of Chicago, Chicago, IL, USA

Joshua H. Hou, MD Department of Ophthalmology and Visual Neurosciences, University of Minnesota, Minneapolis, MN, USA

Andrew J. W. Huang, MD, MPH Department of Ophthalmology and Visual Sciences, Washington University, St. Louis, MO, USA

Vincent Michael Imbrogno, DO Contemporary Ophthalmology of Erie, Erie, PA, USA

Johnathan Jeffers, BA University of Chicago Pritzker School of Medicine, Chicago, IL, USA

Clayton Kirk, MD Loyola University Medical Center, Department of Ophthalmology, Maywood, IL, USA

Christine E. Martinez, MD Department of Ophthalmology and Visual Sciences, The Ohio State University, Columbus, OH, USA

Jared J. Murray, MD Department of Ophthalmology and Visual Neurosciences, University of Minnesota, Minneapolis, MN, USA

James J. Reidy, MD, FACS Department of Ophthalmology and Visual Science, The University of Chicago Medicine, Chicago, IL, USA

Lixing W. Reneker, PhD Department of Ophthalmology, University of Missouri, Columbia, MO, USA

Hassan Shah, MD University of Chicago Medical Center, Department of Ophthalmology and Visual Science, Chicago, IL, USA

Megan Silas, MD University of Chicago Medical Center, Department of Ophthalmology and Visual Science, Chicago, IL, USA

Roshni Vasaiwala, MD Loyola University Medical Center, Department of Ophthalmology, Maywood, IL, USA

Anterior Blepharitis

Jared J. Murray and Joshua H. Hou

Introduction

Blepharitis is an inflammatory condition of the eyelid margin that commonly causes varying degrees of erythema, edema, and discomfort. Patients of all ages and ethnic backgrounds are affected. As a single entity, blepharitis is not sight-threatening, but corneal sequelae such as superficial keratopathy, ulceration, and neovascularization can occur. Blepharitis is often divided by experts into anterior and posterior blepharitis. The former involves skin as well as the eyelash base and follicles. Seborrheic and staphylococcal are two common subtypes of anterior blepharitis; this chapter delves into these and others. Posterior blepharitis involves the meibomian glands [1, 2] and is discussed in the following chapter.

Causes of Anterior Blepharitis

Allergic Contact Blepharitis

Allergic contact blepharitis, usually as sequela of contact dermatitis, is caused by a delayed Type IV T-cell hypersensitivity reaction involving one or both eyes. Symptoms commonly develop within 24–72 hours of exposure to ophthalmic medication, environmental substances, or cosmetic products. Frequently implicated ophthalmic medications include cycloplegics, such as atropine and homatropine, and the preservatives thymerosol, ethylenediaminetetraacedic acid (EDTA), and benzalkonium chloride (BAK). Topical aminoglycoside antibiotics (gentamycin, neomycin, and tobramycin) are also routinely implicated [3]. Table 1.1 lists various sources of offending agents.

Classically, patients will complain of intense pruritis. Eyelid erythema and edema are found on exam, often with a scaly eczematous appearance. The conjunctiva may be injected, and depending on the extent, duration, and degree of eye rubbing by the patient, keratopathy may also result. When the

J. J. Murray · J. H. Hou (✉)
Department of Ophthalmology and Visual Neurosciences, University of Minnesota, Minneapolis, MN, USA
e-mail: jhhou@umn.edu

Table 1.1 Sources of allergic dermatoblepharitis [5]

Hand transfer of allergens
Cosmetics: eyelids, face, hair, hands
Topical medications
Makeup brushes and applicators
Objects in contact with the eyelids: eyelash curler, camera eyepiece, goggles, glasses, etc.
Airborne contact dermatitis
Soaps and shampoos
Protein contact dermatitis: dust mites, latex, cornstarch, animal dander, fish, etc.
Metal nail files
Gloves and glove powder
Eye medications and treatments
Dermatitis secondary to blepharitis and conjunctivitis
Plants
Sunscreens
Makeup removers
Artificial nails and nail lacquer
Systemic contact dermatitis
Textiles

condition becomes chronic, ectropion, ptosis, and worsening dermatochalasis can occur. While allergic blepharitis is a common cause of eyelid inflammation, it is often unrecognized by eye care professionals [4].

Atopic Blepharitis

Anterior atopic blepharitis is a common extension or sequela of atopic dermatitis (AD), a chronic inflammatory skin condition. AD has a lifetime prevalence of 15% to 20% effecting both sexes and patients of all ages [6]. The presentation and clinical exam findings of atopic and allergic blepharitis are similar. Patients commonly experience intense itching leading to frequent scratching and rubbing. As with AD, atopic blepharitis is a chronic condition with frequent exacerbations. Disease prevalence ranges from 41% to 53%, with 39.5 to 74.3% developing keratoconjunctivitis [7]. Keratoconus, glaucoma, cataracts, retinal detachments, and herpes simplex virus infections are additional known complications of atopic dermatitis affecting the eyelids. Etiology is likely multifactorial stemming from a combination of genetics, physical trauma from eye rubbing, immune system dysfunction, as well as side effects from atopic dermatitis treatments [7, 8].

Staphylococcal Blepharitis

Blepharitis that is presumed to be infectious in nature is termed staphylococcal blepharitis as *Staphylococcal aureus* is most frequently implicated [1]. Other bacteria may be causative in uncommon cases [1, 9]. Among those diagnosed with staphylococcal or mixed staphylococcal/seborrheic blepharitis, 51% had cultures positive for *S. aureus* compared to 8% of normal eyes [10]. *Staph epidermidis* appears to be ubiquitous but has also been linked to disease. *Propionibacterium acnes*, *Corynebacterium* species, and *Staph epidermidis* have also been found to be more prevalent among diseased eyelids versus controls and there is suggestion that heavy colonization may be a factor. The pathophysiology includes colonization, possible toxin/enzyme-mediated damage, and immune response [9]. Valenton and Okumoto hypothesized that toxins produced by certain strains of *S. aureus* or *S. epidermis* could be pathogenic; however, no toxin has been found in significantly higher association with blepharitic eyelids compared to controls [11, 12].

Staphylococcal blepharitis is especially common among younger patients and manifests with symptoms of burning, itching, foreign-body sensation, and crusting (most-frequently in the morning upon waking). Examination typically reveals hard matted crusts surrounding the anterior eyelid margin cilia. These crusts are referred to as collarettes, of which removal often leads to ulceration. Other exam features include anterior and posterior margin telangiectasias, madarosis, trichiasis, and poliosis. Chronic staphylococcal blepharoconjunctivitis is said to occur when both eyelids and conjunctiva demonstrate pathology with signs and symptoms lasting greater than or equal to 4 weeks. Along with the blepharitis features, the palpebral conjunctiva demonstrates a papillary reaction, especially inferiorly adjacent to the eyelid margin. Both palpebral and bulbar conjunctiva are mildly injected without discharge. *Moraxella lacunata* is associated with angular blepharoconjunctivitis in which focal ulceration of the lateral canthal angle is evident. A follicular or papillary tarsal conjunctival reaction is often present. *Moraxella* blepharoconjunctivitis may present independently, or concomitantly with *S. aureus* blepharoconjunctivitis [1].

Blepharokeratoconjunctivitis (BKC) is a common entity in which various forms of keratitis exist in conjunction with blepharoconjunctivitis. Punctate keratopathy, either diffuse, or inferiorly adjacent to the inferior eyelid margin, is common and can be asymmetric. The most well known associated keratopathy are known as staphylococcal-associated marginal ulcers. These are characterized by one or more gray/white fluffy circular or oval peripheral marginal infiltrates, usually with a small (1 mm or less) area of clear cornea between the infiltrate and limbus (Fig. 1.1). These infiltrates are sterile inflammatory reactions to corneal compromise and antigen. They are often called "catarrhal" ulcers and are commonly located where the eyelid margin and cornea limbus transect (10, 2, 4, and 8 o'clock). Phlyctenules are focal hyperemic inflammatory nodules of the cornea or conjunctiva. In developed countries, they are frequently associated with *Staphylococcal aureus*. In tuberculosis-endemic regions of the world, phlyctenules are associated with *Mycobacterium tuberculosis* infections among malnourished children. Prior studies suggest that both phlyctenulosis and staphylococcal-associated marginal keratitis (catarrhal keratopathy) develop from cell-mediated delayed hypersensitivity reaction to the cell wall of *S. aureus* [1, 13, 14]. The peripheral cornea's location near limbal vasculature and conjunctival lymphoid tissue make it susceptible to immunologic reactivity [14].

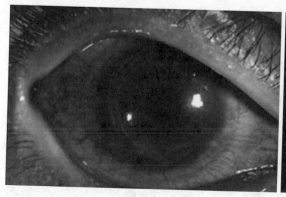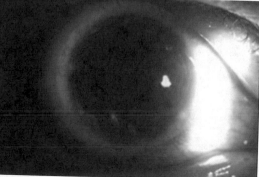

Fig. 1.1 Staphylococcal blepharokeratoconjunctivitis with marginal ("catarrhal") ulcers. (From Guin [5], with permission of Elsevier)

Seborrheic Blepharitis

Seborrheic blepharitisis is an inflammatory condition primarily involving the anterior eyelid margin that tends to disproportionally affect older patients without a gender disparity. Variable amounts of oily/greasy scaling or scurf on the eyelids and/or lashes is characteristic on slit lamp examination (Fig. 1.2). Seborrheic blepharitis often occurs in conjunction with seborrheic dermatitis, in which case, similar debris is usually present in the eyebrows and scalp. Many patients will also have Meibomian gland disease (MGD) evidenced by over-secretion of turbid-appearing oil from gland orifices can be expressed on exam. Like other forms of blepharitis, eyelid redness is common. Approximately 15% of patients develop keratitis, typically across the lower one third of the cornea in the way of punctate epithelial erosions, and 30% have evaporative dry eye disease [1]. Not surprisingly, patients commonly experience burning, eye dryness, and foreign-body sensation.

Demodex Blepharitis

When eyelash sleeves are noted on exam with other signs and symptoms persisting despite consistent conventional blepharitis treatment, demodicosis should be suspected [1].The cylindrical sleeve-like dandruff particles frequently found with this type of blepharitis harbor mites. Interestingly, neither the number of mites or nor the extent of dandruff has been shown to correlate with symptom severity. Two different *Demodex* species are known to cause blepharitis, *Demodex folliculorum* and *Demodex brevis*. *D. folliculorum* measures 0.3–0.4 mm, is found at lash roots and follicles, and is specifically associated with anterior blepharitis (Fig. 1.3). *D. brevis* measures slightly smaller at 0.2–0.3 mm, is found in sebaceous and meibomian glands, and is a known cause of posterior blepharitis, meibomian gland dysfunction, recurrent chalazia, and treatment refractory keratoconjunctivitis [15]. *D. folliculorum* is found more frequently than *D. brevis* in ocular infestation. Prevalence of both species increases with age [16].

The *Demodex* mite life cycle runs approximately 14–18 days and includes egg, larval, and adult stages. Demodex mites require a living host and trans-infestation requires direct contact. Various pathological changes have been implicated during demodicosis of the eyelids. First, physical blockage of follicles with reactive hyperkeratinization and epithelial hyperplasia is common. The parasite may also serve as a vector for bacteria (typically *Bacillus oleronius)* acting as a co-pathogen [17]. Parasite chitin itself may cause an inflammatory foreign body reaction. Finally, the presence of mites and their waste products may stimulate humoral and cell-mediated immune reactions [18].

Fig. 1.2 Seborrheic blepharitis

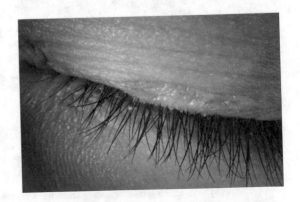

Fig. 1.3 *Demodex folliculorum*

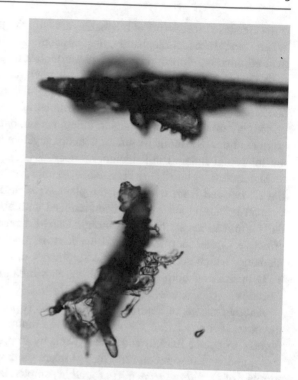

Demodex prevalence has been shown to be widespread, even among normal adults without blepharitis. For this reason, uniform diagnosis standards are lacking, including criteria for number of eyelashes sampled and number of mites identified. In vivo confocal microscopy (IVCM) appears to be more accurate diagnostically than examining eyelashes with light microscopy. IVCM can effectively identify a single mite on a single lash, but identification may be limited by investigator experience [19].

Treatment

When allergic blepharitis is suspected, identifying and discontinuing exposure to the offending agent are the critical first steps in management. Cool compresses, as well as systemic (diphenhydramine, cetirizine) and topical (ketotifen) antihistamine medications can help with pruritus. Topical mast cell-stabilizing treatment with olopatadine or cromolyn can also be helpful [3].

Treatment of atopic blepharitis is grounded in lid hygiene, including warm compresses and gentle eyelid cleansing with baby shampoo and over-the-counter cleansing pads. Topical steroids are often used for treatment of flare-ups, but their adverse side effects (increased intraocular pressure (IOP) and glaucoma, subcapsular cataract, herpes simplex reactivation, and skin atrophy), limit long-term, chronic use [20]. Calcineurin inhibitors, such as cyclosporin, and the macrolide tacrolimus have immunomodulatory effects that have been shown to be beneficial in the treatment of posterior and anterior blepharitis. Tacrolimus acts as an immunosuppressant by inhibiting transcription activity through the nuclear factor of activated T cells' (NFAT) pathway. Topical tacrolimus has been used to treat atopic dermatitis skin lesions since 2001 [7]. Topical use in the treatment of belpharoconjunctivitis has been shown to be efficacious and safe in the long term [20].

Warm compresses and eyelid hygiene are nearly universal staples for treatment of staphylococcal, seborrheic, and demodex blepharitis. Tear film insufficiency generally improves with use of artificial tears. Because most forms of blepharitis are chronic, these measures need to be continued long term. When staphylococcal blepharitis, blepharoconjunctivitis, or BKC is in question, eyelid and conjunctival cultures are appropriate. Topical antibiotics (erythromycin, bacitracin, etc.) are used regularly with the goal of reducing bacterial load; however, frequent use has led to microbial resistance. Combination antibiotic/corticosteroids are popular for conveniently treating bacterial colonization and quieting inflammation as a single treatment. In combination or when used alone, topical steroids effectively treat flare-up-associated inflammation, but patients must be monitored for steroid-related complications. Systemic treatment with doxycycline or azithromycin may be beneficial for both their antimicrobial and anti-inflammatory properties [20].

Demodex blepharitis has been shown to improve with treatment using tea tree oil (TTO), an essential oil derived from the leaf of the plant *Melaleuca alternifolia*. Eyelid margin, conjunctival, and corneal inflammation have all been reduced with 50% TTO application weekly in clinic plus 10% daily applications at home for 1 month. Daily lid massage with 5% TTO at home has also been found effective. Contact dermatitis may occur due to terpinolene, α-terpinene, ascaridole, and 1,2,4-trihydroxy methane, which are found in TTO. Terpinen-4-ol is possibly the most effective active ingredient in TTO possessing both antimicrobial and anti-inflammatory properties and is the sole ingredient in Cliradex® (Bio-Tissue, Inc.) [21].

Another means of controlling demodicosis is prevention of physical transfer from one follicle to the next. Mercury oxide 1% ointment, sulfur ointment, pilocarpine gel, and camphorated oil applied nightly to eyelid margin and lashes work by trapping mites. Both topical ivermectin 1% applied daily, and oral ivermectin (200 μg/kg) taken on day 0 and day 7 have been reported to reduce the number of *D. folliculorum* mites found in sampled lashes [17, 21].

With chronic unilateral blepharitis, particularly in the presence of madarosis and lid thickening, malignancies such as squamous cell, basal cell, and especially sebaceous cell carcinoma, must be ruled out. When symptoms persist with one eye only, nasolacrimal duct obstruction should be considered. When one or both eyes are affected chronically without treatment response, susceptibility testing may be useful to guide antimicrobial treatment. Demodex and factitious etiologies should be considered when clinical improvement is not evident despite treatment [1].

Compliance with Ethical Requirements Jared Murray and Joshua H. Hou declare that they have no conflict of interest. No human or animal studies were carried out by the authors for this chapter.

References

1. Weisenthal RW, Daly MK, de Freitas D, editors. American Academy of ophthalmology basic clinical science course: external disease and cornea. Vol. 8. San Francisco: American Academy of Ophthalmology; 2018–2019;69–77.
2. Lindsley K, Matsumura S, Hatef E, Akpek EK. Interventions for chronic blepharitis. Cochrane Database Syst Rev. 2012;2012(5):CD005556. https://doi.org/10.1002/14651858.CD005556.pub2. PMID: 22592706; PMCID: PMC4270370
3. Shaw SS, Oetting TO. Allergic contact dermatoblepharitis. https://webeye.ophth.uiowa.edu/eyeforum/cases/80-Dermatoblepharitis.htm. Accessed Dec 1, 2019.
4. Chishom SAM, Couch SM, Custer PL. Etiology and management of allergic eyelid dermatitis. Ophthal Plast Reconstr Surg. 2017;33:248–50.
5. Guin JD. Eyelid dermatitis: experience in 203 cases. J Am Acad Dermatol. 2002;47(5):755–65.
6. Hsu JI, Pflugfelder SC, Kim SJ. Ocular complications of atopic dermatitis. Cutis. 2019;104(03):189–93.
7. Yamamoto K, Wakabyashi Y, Kawakami S, et al. Recent trends of ocular complications in patients with atopic dermatitis. Jpn J Ophthalmol. 2019;63(5):410–6. https://doi.org/10.1007/s10384-019-00678-3. Epub 2019 Jun 26
8. Govind K, Whang K, Khanna R, et al. Atopic dermatitis is associated with increased prevalence of multiple ocular comorbidities. J Allergy Clin Immunol Pract. 2019;7(1):298–9. https://doi.org/10.1016/j.jaip.2018.10.009. Epub 2018 Oct 17

9. Jackson WB. Blepharitis: current strategies for diagnosis and management. Can J Ophthalmol. 2008;43(2):170–9. https://doi.org/10.1139/i08-016.

10. Dougherty JM, McCulley JP. Comparative bacteriology of chronic blepharitis. Br J Ophthalmol. 1984;68(8):524–8.

11. Valenton MJ, Okumoto M. Toxin-producing strains of *Staphylococcus epidermidis* (albus). Isolates from patients with staphylococcic blepharoconjunctivitis. Arch Ophthalmol. 1973;89(3):186–9.

12. Seal D, Ficker L, Ramakrishnan M, Wright P. Role of staphylococcal toxin production in blepharitis. Ophthalmology. 1990;97(12):1684–8.

13. Boto-de-los-Bueis A, del Hierro Zarzuelo A, García Perea A, de Pablos M, Pastora N, Noval S. *Staphylococcus aureus* blepharitis associated with multiple corneal stromal microabscess, stromal edema, and uveitis. Ocul Immunol Inflamm. 2015;23(2):180–3. https://doi.org/10.3109/09273948.2013.870214.

14. Kaufman SCAR, Allison E. Peripheral corneal disease. In: CORNEA, fundamentals, diagnosis, and management. Maryland Heights, MO: Elsevier; 2017; chapter 19. p. 232–40.

15. Cheng AM, Sheha H, Tseng SDC. Recent advances on ocular Demodex infestation. Current Opin Ophthalmol. 2015;26(4):295–300. ISSN:1040-8738, 1531-7021. https://doi.org/10.1097/ICU.0000000000000168.

16. Moris García V, Valenzuela Vargas G, Marín Cornuy M, Aguila Torres P. Ocular demodicosis: A review. Arch Soc Esp Oftalmol. 2019;94(7):316–22. https://doi.org/10.1016/j.oftal.2019.04.003. Epub 2019 May 29.

17. Litwin D, Chen W, Dzika E, Korycinska J. Human permanent ectoparasites; recent advances on biology and clinical significance of demodex mites: narrative review article. Iran J Parasitol. 2017;12(1):12–21.

18. Czepita D, Kuźna-Grygiel W, Czepita M, Grobelny A. Demodexfolliculorum and Demodex brevis as a cause of chronic marginal blepharitis. Ann Acad Med Stetin. 2007;53(1):63–7. discussion 67

19. Yang YJ, Ke M, Chen XM. Prospective study of the diagnostic accuracy of the in vivo scanning confocal microscopy for ocular Demodicosis. Am J Ophthalmol. 2019;203:46–52.

20. Kiiski V, Remitz A, Reitamo S, Mandelin J, Kari O. Long-term safety of topical pimecrolimus and topical tacrolimus in atopicblepharoconjunctivitis. JAMA Dermatol. 2014;150(5):571–3.

21. Sabeti S, Kheirkhah A, Yin J, Dana R. Management of meibomian gland dysfunction: a review. Surv Ophthalmol. 2020;65(2):205–17. https://doi.org/10.1016/j.survophthal.2019.08.007. Epub 2019 Sep 5

Posterior Blepharitis

2

Christine E. Martinez, Lixing W. Reneker, and Andrew J. W. Huang

Introduction and Definition

Blepharitis is a chronic inflammatory condition of the eyelids, which can affect ocular surface integrity and lead to ocular irritation and discomfort. Based on anatomical location, blepharitis can be classified as anterior or posterior. Posterior blepharitis is a heterogeneous condition defined as lid margin inflammation posterior to the gray line and may include the following structures: the marginal mucosa, mucocutaneous junction, meibomian glands, and neighboring keratinized skin. Meibomian gland dysfunction (MGD) is one cause of posterior blepharitis and with increasing frequency the two terms are used synonymously [1]. However, there are other etiologies of posterior blepharitis such as infectious or allergic blepharoconjunctivitis, so it is more accurate to consider these conditions as separate entities [1]. MGD will be the focus of this chapter.

Meibomian glands are sebaceous glands and their secretory product, meibum, is the primary source of lipids, which constitute the innermost layer of the tear film. Lipid is a critical component of the tear film because it prevents evaporation and enhances tear film stability by lowering the surface tension of tears. The 2011 International Workshop on Meibomian Gland Dysfunction defined MGD as, "*a chronic, diffuse abnormality of the meibomian glands, commonly characterized by terminal duct obstruction and/or qualitative/quantitative changes in the glandular secretion. This may result in alteration of the tear film, symptoms of eye irritation, clinically apparent inflammation, and ocular surface disease*" [1]. MGD may be primary or secondary and can be further subdivided in many ways, including on the basis of low-delivery or high-delivery states. Low delivery of meibomian gland secretions can be caused either by hyposecretion of meibum or obstruction of glandular ducts or orifices [1].

C. E. Martinez (✉)
Department of Ophthalmology and Visual Sciences, The Ohio State University, Columbus, OH, USA

L. W. Reneker
Department of Ophthalmology, University of Missouri, Columbia, MO, USA

A. J. W. Huang
Department of Ophthalmology and Visual Sciences, Washington University, St. Louis, MO, USA

© Springer Nature Switzerland AG 2021
A. V. Farooq, J. J. Reidy (eds.), *Blepharitis*, Essentials in Ophthalmology,
https://doi.org/10.1007/978-3-030-65040-7_2

Dry Eye Association

MGD has a strong association with dry eye disease, which may be primary aqueous deficient, secondary evaporative, or a combination of the two. MGD is thought to be the leading cause of evaporative dry eye [2, 3].

Epidemiology and Risk Factors

To date, no studies have specifically established the epidemiology of posterior blepharitis in general, but a number of population-based studies have sought to determine the prevalence of MGD in particular. The numbers vary widely and reported prevalence ranges from 3.5% in the Salisbury Eye Evaluation study to 69.3% in the Beijing Eye Study [2]. The disparity comes as least in part from lack of consensus on disease-defining characteristics between the studies. Some of the discrepancy can also be accounted for by racial differences, as studies of Asian populations appear to demonstrate higher rates of MGD [2]. Age distribution of the study groups may also play a role in reported disease prevalence because increasing age correlates well with increasing prevalence of MGD.

Hormones

Sex steroids have a major impact on meibomian gland function. Androgens appear to promote meibum secretion and reduce inflammation, while estrogens appear to increase inflammation in meibomian glands in the same manner that other sebaceous glands are affected throughout the body [4]. Androgen deficiency and complete androgen-insensitivity syndrome are each associated with both MGD and tear film instability [2]. Pathologic states that alter androgen action are particularly associated with keratinization of the posterior lid margin and a secondary obstructive MGD [4].

Sex

While it is well known that female sex is a risk factor for dry eye disease [5], the relationship between sex and MGD is less clear [2]. Better tear function in postmenopausal women is associated with higher testosterone levels; however, better tear function in premenopausal women is associated with lower testosterone levels [6]. The effect of menopause on MGD has yet to be elucidated. Meibomian glands in men have a higher expression of particular fatty acid products than age-matched women [5], but it is unclear what role this may play in the pathogenesis of MGD. Men older than 70 years have a higher incidence of lid margin abnormalities and meibomian gland dropout [5].

Age

Aging is a recognized risk factor for MGD. Multiple studies have demonstrated increased signs of MGD with aging, such as lid margin abnormalities and meibomian gland atrophy within the tarsal plate on meibography [2, 7, 8]. Whether this is directly related to normal degenerative changes associated with senescence or is secondary to decreased production of sex-steroid hormones, stem cell diminution, or growth factor deficiency with aging remains unclear. Peroxisome proliferator-activated receptor gamma (PPAR-gamma) is a nuclear receptor protein whose downregulation with increasing age is hypothesized to underlie decreased meibocyte differentiation and lipid synthesis [9, 10].

Medications

Retinoic acid derivatives such as isotretinoin (Accutane), a vitamin A analog, are used in the dermatologic treatment of facial acne and are also components of many anti-aging skin products. 13-cis retinoic acid results in blepharoconjunctivitis, abnormal meibomian secretions, atrophy of meibomian glands, and dry eye signs and symptoms [4, 11]. During treatment with isotretinoin, meibomian glands appear less dense and more atrophic by meibography with an increase in meibum thickness and elevation of tear osmolarity [11]. Additionally, multiple topical medications have been found to alter meibomian gland structure or function. Topical epinephrine causes keratinization of the duct epithelium and subsequent obstructive MGD [12]. Topical glaucoma medications such as beta-blockers, carbonic anhydrase inhibitors, and prostaglandin analogs are associated with changes in meibomian gland structure such as decreased acinar area and density and have been associated with MGD in patients on chronic therapy [13, 14].

Systemic Diseases

Rosacea is a chronic inflammatory skin disease characterized by facial erythema and telangiectasia. The disease most commonly affects Caucasians and may cause eyelid and ocular surface inflammation. Compared to age-matched controls, patients with rosacea are more likely to demonstrate lid margin abnormalities, meibomian gland dropout, and decreased density of meibomian glands along the eyelids [15]. Lid margin abnormalities include meibomian orifice retro-placement, lid margin telangiectasia, and rounding or notching of the lid margin. Other systemic disorders have also been associated with posterior blepharitis and these include atopic dermatitis, seborrheic dermatitis, psoriasis, ichthyosis, Sjogren's syndrome, discoid lupus, and ectodermal dysplasia [2]. Posterior blepharitis has also been associated with cicatricial conjunctivitis in diseases such as mucus membrane pemphigoid (MMP), trachoma, erythema multiforme (Stevens-Johnson syndrome), and graft versus host disease (GVHD) [2].

Other

Contact lens wearers have greater degrees of meibomian gland dropout on infrared meibography when compared to age-matched controls who do not wear contact lenses [16]. Young contact lens wearers have been observed to have a meibomian gland dropout rate similar to individuals in their 60's with age-related glandular degeneration [16]. Arita et al. found that the duration of contact lens wear was also positively correlated with extent of meibomian gland dropout. This suggests that dry eye associated with contact lens wear may be at least in part related to MGD. One hypothesis for the etiology of meibomian gland dropout is that chronic irritation of the meibomian gland by the contact lens through the conjunctiva causes these pathologic changes.

Smoking may be another risk factor and smokers with MGD have increased lid margin and meibum abnormalities compared to non-smokers with MGD [17].

Anatomy, Etiology, and Pathogenesis

There are 20–30 meibomian glands in the lower eyelid and 25–40 in the upper eyelid [4]. The orifices of the meibomian glands are located just anterior to the mucocutaneus junction, and the normal vertical extent of the glands corresponds roughly to the extent of the respective tarsal plates. Each meibomian gland is composed of secretory acini connected via short ductules to a long central duct. The entire internal system is lined by stratified squamous epithelium with signs of emerging keratinization [4]. Full keratinization is normally only seen in the terminal part of the central duct as it approaches the meibomian gland orifice [4].

Meibum is secreted through a holocrine secretion mechanism and is normally a clear oil, but in MGD it may appear more white or yellow and the consistency may be creamy or like toothpaste. Meibum is composed most abundantly of wax, fatty acids and fatty alcohols, cholesterol, and protein [4]. The transition temperature for meibomian lipids from solid to liquid ranges from 28 to 32 degrees Celsius, and therefore eyelid temperature will affect the viscosity of meibum [4].The meibum is secreted onto the eyelid margin under both neural and hormonal control and is aided by blinking. During sleep the meibum is thought to accumulate in the glands near the orifices and with waking and recommencement of blinking, the excess is discharged from the glands [18].

Pathogenesis

The pathophysiology of posterior blepharitis and MGD is complex and likely multifactorial. Hyperkeratinization of ductal epithelium has been considered to be an important cause of obstructive MGD and is influenced by a variety of factors such as advancing age, hormonal abnormalities, medication toxicity, and contact lens wear [4]. The secretory ducts then become plugged and obstructed by desquamated epithelial cells and thickened, viscous meibum. Progressively the ducts then become dilated secondary to accumulation of meibum, and subsequently there is secondary loss of secretory meibocytes [4]. This process results in diminished delivery of meibum to the tear film and ocular surface. Meibomian gland obstruction is probably the most common form of MGD [1].

Atrophy and degeneration of the glandular acini may result in a secondary hyposecretion [4]. Meibomian gland dropout has been correlated with decreased meibum production [19]. Atrophy may be caused by increased intraglandular pressure secondary to obstruction and meibum stasis, and this may inhibit normal cell differentiation. Eventually the short ductules and subsequently the acini undergo squamous metaplasia that results in keratinization of the epithelium of the ducts and acini. The meibomian gland orifices also narrow. There is also evidence that atrophy is a primary process in some individuals and may be related to advancing age [4]. Histology of atrophic meibomian glands demonstrates decreased acini size, irregular acini shape, and basement membrane thickening [4]. Corroborative with the above notions, a recent histopathological study, based on a small sample size, suggests potentially distinct pathogenic mechanisms in MGD for patients of different ages. Hyperproliferation and aberrant differentiation of the central ductal epithelia may lead to the obstruction by overproduced cytokeratins in younger adults, whereas decreased cell proliferation in acinar basal epithelia may lead to MG glandular atrophy in older adults [20].

Inflammation

Inflammation, either infectious or noninfectious, can cause posterior blepharitis, but it is not likely an important factor in the development of obstructive MGD [4]. A number of histologic studies have demonstrated granulation tissue with inflammatory cell infiltrate within the meibomian glands of patients with MGD; however, in specimens with ductal dilation and acinar atrophy indicative of obstructive MGD, no inflammatory infiltrate was identified on histology [4]. In vivo confocal microscopy has suggested the possible presence of periglandular inflammatory cells in some individuals with obstructive MGD; however, differentiating between various cell types is difficult with confocal.

Infection

Chronic blepharitis is known to be influenced by overgrowth of commensal bacteria such as coagulase negative staphylococci, *Staphylococcus aureus*, and *Propionibacterium acnes*; however, the role of bacterial infection in MGD is somewhat controversial. Bacterial infection does not appear to play a role in the pathogenesis of obstructive MGD; however, even in the absence of active infection, it is conceivable that bacterial products such as toxins and lipase may play a role in posterior blepharitis [4]. Bacterial lipases and esterases can degrade meibomian lipids resulting in abnormal free fatty acids that may cause inflammation and hyperkeratinization of the lid margin [4]. Oral antibiotics have demonstrated efficacy in the treatment of MGD and posterior blepharitis, but this may have more to do with the anti-inflammatory effects than the antimicrobial effects of these medications [4, 21, 22]. Additionally, *Demodex brevis* mites reside in meibomian glands and may play a role in the pathogenesis of posterior blepharitis [23].

Growth Factors and Cytokines

Fibroblast growth factor receptors (FGFRs) are important for cell differentiation, survival, migration and differentiation. High levels of fibroblast growth factor receptor type 2 (FGFR2) are expressed in the acinar and ductal epithelial cells in meibomian glands of both mice and humans. Deletions of FGFR2 in mice models result in severe meibomian gland acinar atrophy [24]. This suggests that a FGFR2 plays an important role in meibomian gland hemostasis and may be a potential target for novel MGD therapy in the future.

A number of inflammatory tear film cytokines have been associated with MGD. These include IL-4, IL-6, IL-10, IL-17a, and TNF-α [25]. Choi et al. demonstrated decreased levels of these cytokines in the tear film after treatment with intense pulsed light (IPL) therapy. Measurement of inflammatory tear cytokines may serve as an indicator of treatment response in MGD.

Clinical Findings

In normal individuals, the meibomian gland orifices are located just anterior to the mucocutaneous junction and are spaced regularly along the eyelid margins. Clinical findings of posterior blepharitis include eyelid margin telangiectasias, injection, and keratinization. Rounding, notching, dimpling, or scalloping of the posterior lid margin may be observed. Additionally, an epithelial ridge between orifices may be present. Exam findings indicative of MGD also include capping, plugging, or atrophy of the meibomian gland orifices [2]. Manual expression of the glands can demonstrate either excessive or decreased meibum of various characteristics, such as thick or toothpaste-like meibum. The tear film may also be abnormal or unstable, either as a secondary or primary process. In early stages, MGD may be subclinical and asymptomatic, but later it may progress to be both symptomatic and clinically obvious on slit lamp exam.

With chronic posterior blepharitis, the location of the meibomian orifices relative to the mucocutaneous junction may change [18]. The mucocutaneous junction may move anteriorly in the process of conjunctivalization and is thought to represent an aging process. With progression, periductal fibrosis around the meibomian orifices can be visualized. Conversely, in MGD in the setting of cicatricial disease the glands are pulled posteriorly onto the conjunctiva [18]. In this setting, there is stretching and exposure of the terminal ducts that is called ductal exposure. Clinically these orifices appear slightly elevated and rib-like. When periductal fibrosis or ductal exposure is present, these clinical

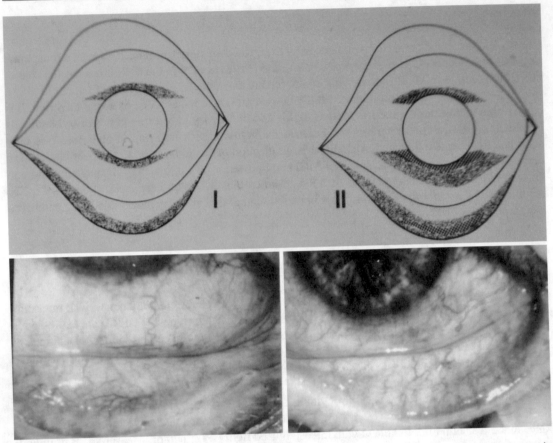

Fig. 2.1 The top images are drawings of classic lid margin and corresponding conjunctival staining patterns seen in posterior blepharitis. The bottom images are representative patient photos demonstrating these staining patterns with rose Bengal.

conditions are thought to be irreversible [18]. Abnormal staining patterns with fluorescein, rose Bengal, or lissamine green may be present. Classically there is staining of the posterior lid margin associated with corresponding staining of the inferior or superior conjunctiva and limbus that are in apposition with the eyelid margins (Fig. 2.1).

Symptoms

MGD has been associated with ocular surface symptoms such as irritation, burning, itching, subjective eye dryness, and teary eyes. It has also been associated with eyelid crusting and stickiness (especially in the morning), eyelid puffiness and heaviness, and both eye and eyelid redness [2]. Notably, these symptoms are similar to those reported in both anterior blepharitis and dry eye disease. Due to abnormal meibum production, MGD may cause evaporative dry eye. Although the pathogenesis of MGD differs from aqueous-deficient dry eye, these two conditions may also co-exist, and it can be difficult to determine whether symptoms are related to MGD, aqueous deficiency, or both [2, 4]. Vision and contrast sensitivity may also be impact by MGD due to tear film instability.

Complications

Posterior blepharitis and MGD are associated with a number of eyelid and ocular surface complications. Chalazia are chronic, granulomatous inflammatory reactions of meibomian glands in the eyelids, and they are generally considered to be noninfectious [26]. Chalazia may arise from internal hordeola, which are acute inflammatory reactions of the meibomian glands that may or may not have an infectious etiology [26]. Both chalazia and internal hordeola are thought to be at least partially related to meibomian gland obstruction and meibum stasis [26]. Blepharitis and acne rosacea are known risk factors for the development of chalazion [15, 26, 27].

Ocular surface disease has also been associated with posterior blepharitis and MGD. This includes conjunctival hyperemia, punctate keratitis, marginal infiltrates, pannus or corneal neovascularization, corneal scar or opacity, phlyctenular keratitis, and peripheral ulcerative keratitis (PUK) (Fig. 2.2) [18, 27, 28]. Proposed mechanisms for these corneal abnormalities include mechanical rubbing of the inflamed eyelid margin, release of inflammatory mediators into the tear film, or consequences of secondary dry eye [18, 27].

Diagnosis

Posterior blepharitis and MGD can be symptomatic and diagnosed on the basis of the clinical findings described previously. MGD can also be an asymptomatic, subclinical condition with subtle or no gross clinical signs. In those cases, it may only be diagnosed with gland expression or additional diagnostic testing. Manual expression of the glands can be performed to determine the color, consistency, and quantity of secretion. Use of a standardized expression device to describe the "expressibility" of the glands has been described [18].

Additional diagnostic tests may be used to further quantify or qualify the disease process, monitor for progression, or confirm the diagnosis. Interferometry can be used to quantify the thickness of the tear film lipid layer, the normal thickness of which is reported to range from 20 to 160 nm [18]. With the upstroke of a blink, the lipid layer can also be seen to spread upwards and then to stabilize. In eyes with lipid deficiency of the tears, the lipid layer is noted to take longer to stabilize [18]. Tear break-up time (TBUT) is a useful tool to evaluate the tear film stability in these patients, and describes the time interval between the last complete blink and the appearance of the first corneal dry spot [3]. A TBUT less than 10 seconds is generally considered abnormal [29].

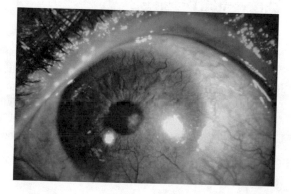

Fig. 2.2 This image demonstrates corneal neovascularization in a patient with meibomian gland dysfunction (MGD). Note the presence of meibomian gland plugging and telangiectasias of the posterior lid margin

Fig. 2.3 The top color photo depicts loss of meibomian gland architecture that is normally visible through the tarsal conjunctiva. The bottom black-and-white photo was taken of the same patient and confirms the loss of normal meibomian glands, which normally appear black in this type of image

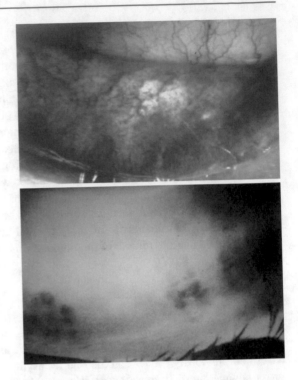

Meibography can be used to assess the architecture of the meibomian glands via transillumination of the eyelids using white light, near infrared, or infrared light (Fig. 2.3). More recently infrared photography and videography with or without transillumination have been utilized in non-contact methods and reported as faster and easier means of obtaining information related to meibomian gland architecture through meibography [2, 8]. The eyelids are everted to obtain the images in all of these techniques. In vivo confocal microscopy has also been used to measure gland diameter through the everted tarsal plate [30].

Meibometry is a technique to quantify the amount of lipid present in the lower lid reservoir and involves blotting a sample of meibum onto a loop of plastic tape [18]. Tests of tear quantity and quality such as TBUT, tear osmolarity, and Schirmer's testing can be used as an indirect measure of meibomian gland dysfunction; however, these tests are generally not specific to MGD [31].

Differential Diagnosis

Chronic allergy with severe ocular inflammation such as atopic keratoconjunctivitis and contact dermatitis due to medications or chemical exposure can often induce severe lid inflammation and mimic MGD or posterior blepharitis. Occasionally, basal cell carcinoma or squamous cell carcinoma can involve the lid margin with secondary MGD. In the presentation of a unilateral blepharoconjunctivitis, sebaceous cell carcinoma arising from meibomian glands or other pilo-sebaceous glands should always be included in the differential diagnosis of MGD. There may be pagetoid spread of the sebaceous cell carcinoma across the bulbar or tarsal conjunctiva [32].

Treatment

Treatment goals of posterior blepharitis are to reduce any present inflammation, improve the flow of meibum, stabilize the tear film, improve ocular comfort, and prevent corneal complications.

Heat and Mechanical Massage

A classic initial treatment for MGD involves application of warmth to the eyelids along with mechanical eyelid massage. Heat application to the eyelids is based on the idea that melting meibum lipids may soften the secretions and improve evacuation of the meibomian glands. The warming has been described and studied in a variety of means, ranging from simple warm compresses to devices such as infrared or hot air sources [21, 33, 34]. In patients treated with daily "eyelid hygiene" consisting of daily eyelid warming, massage, and lid margin scrubbing, one study demonstrated a 5% reversal of meibomian gland dropout [35].

Thermal Pulsation

LipiFlow (TearScience, Morrisville, NC) is an automated, vectored, thermal pulsation system that provides a combination of targeted heat therapy and mechanical massage. The device covers both the back and front of the eyelids. The posterior portion applies heat to the meibomian glands, and the anterior portion gives mechanical stimulation. A recent meta-analysis analyzed the combined outcomes of 4 randomized controlled trials on the efficacy of a single treatment with LipiFlow followed by daily warm compresses for the treatment of MGD [34]. All of the studies included were determined by the authors to be at high risk for inclusion of some type of bias. Improvement in TBUT and a standardized subjective dry-eye score was observed at 2–4 weeks; however, this effect was not sustained at 3 months. Standardized Patient Evaluation of Eye Dryness (SPEED) scores were noted to improve at 2–4 weeks in the treatment group compared to the control group, but this effect was lost at 3 months. There was no change in ocular surface staining pattern, tear osmolarity, Schirmer's test, or lipid layer thickness at any time interval. Ocular Surface Disease Index (OSDI) score was the only metric noted to be improved in the treatment group at both 2–4 weeks and 3 months [34]. This suggests that LipiFlow may not have a lasting therapeutic effect. Providers interested in offering this treatment modality could consider repeating it every 1–2 months.

Intense Pulsed Light (IPL) Therapy

IPL is an accepted, effective, and well-tolerated treatment for a range of dermatologic conditions including hypertrichosis, port wine stains, and telangiectasias [36]. IPL combined with meibomian gland expression has been shown to improve both objective signs and subjective symptoms for a broad range of patients with MGD, including those with severe, refractory MGD [37]. The mechanism of improvement in MGD is likely related to the heating of the eyelid and subsequent melting of the meibum. Hemoglobin absorption of light may also account for decreased lid margin telangiectasias [37].

Mechanical Expression of Meibum

Expression of the meibomian glands to relieve and remove ductal obstructions has been described for over 100 years [38]. Simple manual methods have been described and more recently an instrument called the "Meibomian Gland Squeezer" was found to improve both signs and symptoms of MGD at 1 month [38]. All of the patients in that study reported at least mild pain with the treatment.

Meibomian Gland Probing

In view of the obstructive nature of MGD in many patients, meibomian gland probing has been proposed as a treatment method and a means of restoring intraductal integrity. The theory behind this treatment is that the cycle of meibum stasis and subsequent glandular atrophy can be improved if orifice obstructions that prevent normal meibum expression can be mitigated. One study examined the impact of probing the glands of individuals with refractory MGD with a special cannula. At 3 months, there was an improvement in the OSDI score, an increase in the tear break-up time (TBUT), and a decrease in both conjunctival injection and eyelid margin vascularization [39].

A recent study involving gland probing with a 1 mm intraductal probe demonstrated mechanical resistance to probing in 84% of glands [40]. Of the glands that demonstrated resistance, 79.5% of them were classified as fixed, firm, focal, unyielding resistance (FFFUR) consistent with presumed findings of periglandular fibrosis by confocal microscopy. The probe findings suggest that obstruction of meibomian gland orifices in patients with MGD may be related to more chronic and permanent changes than mere plugging and keratinization.

Artificial Tears and Lipid Supplements

Artificial lubricants are often used to treat concomitant dry eye in patients with MGD [3]. Topical lipid supplements in the form of 2% castor oil drops have demonstrated improved signs and symptoms of MGD [41]. Oral supplementation with omega-3 fatty acids in patients with MGD may improve both tear film stability and contrast sensitivity [42]. Improved contrast sensitivity likely correlates to improved ocular surface and tear film stability. Omega-3 fatty acids are known to be anti-inflammatory as opposed to omega-6 fatty acids, which are proinflammatory. While the study did not specifically distinguish MGD from aqueous tear deficiency, a recent well-controlled trial known as Dry Eye Assessment and Management (DREAM) Research showed omega-3 fatty acid supplements taken orally proved no better than placebo at relieving symptoms or signs of dry eye [43].

Antibiotics

In the United States, oral azithromycin and tetracyclines such as tetracycline, doxycycline, and minocycline are commonly used off-label for treatment of MGD. The efficacy of the tetracyclines is thought to be primarily due to their anti-inflammatory action; however, their antibacterial impact on the commensal eyelid species may also play a role [44]. The tetracycline family is bacteriostatic and have been shown to decrease the production of bacterial lipases, modulate neutrophil and lymphocyte function, and inhibit inflammatory cytokines such as TNF-alpha, MMP-8, and MMP-9 [21]. There are many studies on the use of tetracyclines for MGD; however, very few of them are randomized control trials. One study of 60 patients comparing the use of oral minocycline demonstrated improvement in all signs and symptoms of MGD that were measured in the study [45]. Typically prescribed doses of doxycycline and minocycline are 50-100 mg once or twice per day. At these doses, it is thought that the anti-inflammatory effect plays a larger role than the antibiotic effect on the ocular surface. Patients should be forewarned about the potential side effects of systemic tetracyclines such as skin photosensitivity and gastric irritation. Tetracyclines should be avoided in pediatric patients due to the risk of tooth discoloration [46].

Azithromycin, a macrolide antibiotic, reduces growth of eyelid bacteria, suppresses bacterial lipases, and improves conjunctival inflammation by decreasing the release of proinflammatory molecules [21]. Additionally and uniquely, azithromycin directly stimulates meibomian gland epithelial cells in humans and increases cellular levels of many components of meibum [44]. Multiple studies have demonstrated improvement in signs and symptoms of MGD when treated with oral azithromycin [47]. Yildiz et al. demonstrated improvement in OSDI score, lissamine green staining, and Schirmer's test results with both oral and topical azithromycin in patients with posterior blepharitis [48]. In this study, topical azithromycin also improved TBUT. Topical azithromycin has also been shown to decrease proinflammatory mediators in the tear film [49]. Typically prescribed doses of oral azithromycin for posterior blepharitis are 500 mg to 1 g per day for 1–3 days at a time [47]. Azithromycin may be prescribed in a pulsed fashion because of its long half-life. A one-time oral dose of 1 g of azithromycin maintains its minimum inhibitory concentration (MIC) of 0.25 µg/mL for *Staphylococcus aureus* for 4 days in tears and 14 days in conjunctiva [47].

Oral and topical metronidazole have been reported as treatment modalities for blepharoconjunctvitis in rosacea, both in adult and pediatric populations [27]. Topical metronidazole improves clinical signs of oculocutaneous rosacea compared to placebo [50]. Oral and topical metronidazole have also been studied for the treatment of Demodex blepharitis, but in a recent meta-analysis neither treatment was found to improve the eradication rate of mites or patient-reported symptoms [23].

Tea Tree Oil

Topical tea tree oil and terpinen-4-ol are also used to treat Demodex blepharitis. Based on results of the same recent meta-analysis, both treatments decrease mite counts, improve eradication rates, and improve symptoms [23].

Anti-Inflammatory Agents

Cyclosporine A is an immunosuppressive medication with anti-inflammatory properties that has gained popularity in a dilute topical formulation for the treatment of dry eye conditions. Interestingly, topical 0.05% cyclosporine A has also been shown to improve signs, but not symptoms, of posterior blepharitis [51].

Tacrolimus is a macrolide with immunomodulatory effects and a similar mechanism of action to that of cyclosporine; however, it is 10 to 100 times more potent. Compared to placebo, 0.03% tacrolimus ointment was effective for treatment of signs of posterior blepharitis including improvement in fluorescein staining, rose Bengal staining, eyelid margin telangiectasias, and meibomian gland secretion [52]. However, there was no statistical difference between the treatment and control groups in terms of symptoms studied.

Lifitegrast is a T-cell antagonist that prevents the release of proinflammatory cytokines. It has demonstrated efficacy in the treatment of dry eye disease, but to date there have been no studies examining its role in the treatment of patients with posterior blepharitis [21].

Topical steroids are efficacious in the management of acute inflammation associated with posterior blepharitis and associated corneal complications; however, there are currently no published studies to support the long-term and efficacious use of topical steroids for MGD [21]. In noninfectious MGD, judicious pulsed therapy of topical steroids to suppress the ocular surface inflammation may be warranted.

Future Horizons

Although the literature is ripe with studies on MGD, there is limited understanding of its pathogenesis and effective therapeutic strategies. Future work should focus on elucidating the role of inflammation in MGD more definitively as well as the underlying cellular and molecular mechanisms of MGD and glandular homeostasis. These efforts will aid in the development of targeted therapies for MGD and regenerative medicine for involutional MG atrophy.

Compliance with Ethical Requirements

Conflict of Interest
Christine Martinez, Andrew Huang, and Lixing Reneker declare that they have no conflict of interest.

Informed Consent
No human studies were carried out by the authors for this chapter.

Animal Studies
No animal studies were carried out by the authors for this chapter.

Citations

1. Daniel Nelson J, Shimazaki J, Benitez-del-Castillo JM, Craig J, McCulley JP, Den S, et al. The international workshop on meibomian gland dysfunction: report of the definition and classification subcommittee. Investig Ophthalmol Vis Sci. 2011;52(4):1930–7.
2. Schaumberg DA, Nichols JJ, Papas EB, Tong L, Uchino M, Nichols KK. The international workshop on meibomian gland dysfunction: report of the subcommittee on the epidemiology of, and associated risk factors for. MGD Investig Ophthalmol Vis Sci. 2011;52(4):1994–2005.
3. Vu CHV, Kawashima M, Yamada M, Suwaki K, Uchino M, Shigeyasu C, et al. Influence of Meibomian gland dysfunction and friction-related disease on the severity of dry eye. Ophthalmology [Internet]. 2018;125(8):1181–8. Available from: https://doi.org/10.1016/j.ophtha.2018.01.025
4. Knop E, Knop N, Millar T, Obata H, Sullivan DA. The international workshop on meibomian gland dysfunction: report of the subcommittee on anatomy, physiology, and pathophysiology of the meibomian gland. Investig Ophthalmol Vis Sci. 2011;52(4):1938–78.
5. Sullivan DA, Rocha EM, Aragona P, Clayton JA, Ding J, Golebiowski B, et al. TFOS DEWS II sex, gender, and hormones report. Ocul Surf [Internet]. 2017;15(3):284–333. Available from:. https://doi.org/10.1016/j.jtos.2017.04.001.
6. Mathers WD, Stovall D, Lane JA, Zimmerman MB, Johnson S. Menopause and tear function: the influence of prolactin and sex hormones on human tear production. Cornea. 1998;17(4):353–8.
7. Alghamdi YA, Mercado C, McClellan AL, Batawi H, Karp CL, Galor A. Epidemiology of meibomian gland dysfunction in an elderly population. Cornea. 2016;35(6):731–5.
8. Arita R, Itoh K, Inoue K, Amano S. Noncontact infrared meibography to document age-related changes of the Meibomian glands in a normal population. Ophthalmology. 2008;115(5):911–5.
9. Hwang HS, Parfitt GJ, Brown DJ, Jester JV. Meibocyte differentiation and renewal: insights into novel mechanisms of meibomian gland dysfunction (MGD). Exp Eye Res. 2017;163:37–45.
10. Chhadva P, Goldhardt R, Galor A. Meibomian gland disease: the role of gland dysfunction in dry eye disease. Ophthalmology [Internet]. 2017;124(11):S20–6. Available from: https://doi.org/10.1016/j.ophtha.2017.05.031

11. Mathers WD, Shields WJ, Sachdev MS, Petroll M, Jester JV. Meibomian gland morphology and tear osmolarity: changes with Accutane therapy. Cornea. 1991;10(4):286–90.

12. Jester JV, Nicolaides N, Kiss-Palvolgyi I, Smith RE. Meibomian gland dysfunction. II. The role of keratinization in a rabbit model of MGD. Investig Ophthalmol Vis Sci. 1989;30(5):936–45.

13. Uzunosmanoglu E, Mocan MC, Kocabeyoglu S, Karakaya J, Irkec M. Meibomian gland dysfunction in patients receiving long-term glaucoma medications. Cornea. 2016;35(8):1112–6.

14. Agnifili L, Fasanella V, Costagliola C, Ciabattoni C, Mastropasqua R, Frezzotti P, et al. In vivo confocal microscopy of meibomian glands in glaucoma. Br J Ophthalmol. 2013;97(3):343–9.

15. Machalińska A, Zakrzewska A, Markowska A, Safranow K, Wiszniewska B, Parafiniuk M, et al. Morphological and functional evaluation of Meibomian gland dysfunction in Rosacea patients. Curr Eye Res [Internet]. 2016;41(8):1029–34. Available from:. https://doi.org/10.3109/02713683.2015.1088953.

16. Arita R, Itoh K, Inoue K, Kuchiba A, Yamaguchi T, Amano S. Contact Lens Wear is associated with decrease of Meibomian glands. Ophthalmology. 2009;116(3):379–84.

17. Wang S, Zhao H, Huang C, Li Z, Li W, Zhang X, et al. Impact of chronic smoking on meibomian gland dysfunction. PLoS One. 2016;11(12):1–8.

18. Tomlinson A, Bron AJ, Korb DR, Amano S, Paugh JR, Ian Pearce E, et al. The international workshop on Meibomian gland dysfunction: report of the diagnosis subcommittee. Investig Ophthalmol Vis Sci. 2011;52(4):2006–49.

19. Adil MY, Xiao J, Olafsson J, Chen X, Lagali NS, Ræder S, et al. Meibomian gland morphology is a sensitive early indicator of Meibomian gland dysfunction. Am J Ophthalmol [Internet]. 2019;200:16–25. Available from: https://doi.org/10.1016/j.ajo.2018.12.006

20. Reneker LW, Irlmeier RT, Shui YB, Liu Y, Huang AJW. Histopathology and selective biomarker expression in human meibomian glands. Br J Ophthalmol. 2019:1–6.

21. Sabeti S, Kheirkhah A, Yin J, Dana R. Management of Meibomian gland dysfunction: a review. Surv Ophthalmol [Internet]. 2019:1–13. Available from: https://doi.org/10.1016/j.survophthal.2019.08.007

22. Liu Y, Ding J. The combined effect of azithromycin and insulin-like growth Factor-1 on cultured human Meibomian gland. IOVS. 2014;55(9):5596–601.

23. Navel V, Mulliez A, Benoist d'Azy C, Baker JS, Malecaze J, Chiambaretta F, et al. Efficacy of treatments for Demodex blepharitis: a systematic review and meta-analysis. Ocul Surf. 2019;17(4):655–69.

24. Reneker LW, Wang L, Irlmeier RT, Huang AJW. Fibroblast growth factor receptor 2 (FGFR2) is required for meibomian gland homeostasis in the adult mouse. Investig Ophthalmol Vis Sci. 2017;58(5):2638–46.

25. Choi M, Han SJ, Ji YW, Choi YJ, Jun I, Alotaibi MH, et al. Meibum expressibility improvement as a therapeutic target of intense pulsed light treatment in Meibomian gland dysfunction and its association with tear inflammatory cytokines. Sci Rep [Internet]. 2019;9(1):1–8. Available from:. https://doi.org/10.1038/s41598-019-44000-0.

26. Nemet AY, Vinker S, Kaiserman I. Associated morbidity of chalazia. Cornea. 2011;30(12):1376–81.

27. Suzuki T, Teramukai S, Kinoshita S. Meibomian glands and ocular surface inflammation. Ocul Surf. 2015;13(2):133–49.

28. Sharma N, Sinha G, Shekhar H, Titiyal JS, Agarwal T, Chawla B, et al. Demographic profile, clinical features and outcome of peripheral ulcerative keratitis: a prospective study. Br J Ophthalmol. 2015;99(11):1503–8.

29. Qazi Y, Kheirkhah A, Blackie C, Trinidad M, Williams C, Cruzat A, et al. Clinically relevant immune-cellular metrics of inflammation in Meibomian gland dysfunction. Investig Ophthalmol Vis Sci. 2018;59(15):6111–23.

30. Geerling G, Baudouin C, Aragona P, Rolando M, Boboridis KG, Benítez-del-Castillo JM, et al. Emerging strategies for the diagnosis and treatment of Meibomian gland dysfunction: proceedings of the OCEAN group meeting. Ocul Surf. 2017;15(2):179–92.

31. Giannaccare G, Vigo L, Pellegrini M, Sebastiani S, Carones F. Ocular surface workup with automated noninvasive measurements for the diagnosis of Meibomian gland dysfunction. Cornea. 2018;37(6):740–5.

32. Sawada Y, Fischer JL, Verm AM, Harrison AR, Yuan C, Huang AJW. Detection by impression cytologic analysis of conjunctival intraepithelial invasion from eyelid sebaceous cell carcinoma. Ophthalmology. 2003;110(10):2045–50.

33. Geerling G, Tauber J, Baudouin C, Goto E, Matsumoto Y, O'Brien T, et al. The international workshop on meibomian gland dysfunction: report of the subcommittee on management and treatment of Meibomian gland dysfunction. Investig Ophthalmol Vis Sci. 2011;52(4):2050–64.

34. Pang S-P, Chen Y-T, Tam K-W, Lin I-C, Loh E-W. Efficacy of vectored thermal pulsation and warm compress treatments in Meibomian gland dysfunction. Cornea. 2019;38(6):690–7.

35. Yin Y, Gong L. Reversibility of gland dropout and significance of eyelid hygiene treatment in Meibomian gland dysfunction. Cornea. 2017;36(3):332–7.

36. Raulin C, Greve B, Grema H. IPL technology: a review. Lasers Surg Med. 2003;32(2):78–87.

37. Arita R, Mizoguchi T, Fukuoka S, Morishige N. Multicenter study of intense pulsed light therapy for patients with refractory Meibomian gland dysfunction. Cornea. 2018;37(12):1566–71.

38. Wang DH, Liu XQ, Hao XJ, Zhang YJ, Zhu HY, Dong ZG. Effect of the Meibomian gland squeezer for treatment of Meibomian gland dysfunction. Cornea. 2018;37(10):1270–8.

39. Sarman ZS, Cucen B, Yuksel N, Cengiz A, Caglar Y. Effectiveness of intraductal Meibomian gland probing for obstructive meibomian gland dysfunction. Cornea. 2016;35(6):721–4.

40. Maskin SL, Alluri S. Expressible Meibomian glands have occult fixed obstructions: findings from Meibomian gland probing to restore intraductal integrity. Cornea. 2019;38(7):880–7.

41. Goto E, Shimazaki J, Monden YU, Takano Y, Yagi Y, Shimmura S, et al. Low-concentration homogenized castor oil eye drops for noninflamed obstructive meibomian gland dysfunction. Ophthalmology. 2002;109(11):2030–5.

42. Malhotra C, Singh S, Chakma P, Jain AK. Effect of oral omega-3 fatty acid supplementation on contrast sensitivity in patients with moderate meibomian gland dysfunction: a prospective placebo-controlled study. Cornea. 2015;34(6):637–43.

43. Asbell PA, Maguire G, Pistilli M, Ying GS, Szczotka-Flynn LB, Hardten DR, et al. n−3 Fatty acid supplementation for the treatment of dry eye disease. N Engl J Med. 2018;378(18):1681–90.

44. Liu Y, Kam W, Ding J, Sullivan D. Can tetracycline antibiotics duplicate the ability of azithromycin to stimulate human meibomian gland epithelial cell differentiation? Cornea. 2015;34:342–6.

45. Lee H, Min K, Kim EK, Kim TI. Minocycline controls clinical outcomes and inflammatory cytokines in moderate and severe Meibomian gland dysfunction. Am J Ophthalmol. 2012;154(6):949–957.e1.

46. Wormser GP, Wormser RP, Strle F, Myers R, Cunha BA. How safe is doxycycline for young children or for pregnant or breastfeeding women? Diagn Microbiol Infect Dis [Internet]. 2019;93(3):238–42. Available from: https://doi.org/10.1016/j.diagmicrobio.2018.09.015

47. Igami TZ, Holzchuh R, Osaki TH, Santo RM, Kara-jose N, Hida RY. Oral azithromycin for treatment of posterior blepharitis. Cornea. 2011;30(10):1145–9.

48. Yildiz E, Yenerel NM, Turan-Yardimci A, Erkan M, Gunes P. Comparison of the clinical efficacy of topical and systemic azithromycin treatment for posterior blepharitis. J Ocul Pharmacol Ther. 2018;34(4):365–72.

49. Zhang L, Su Z, Zhang Z, Lin J, Li D-Q, Pflugfelder SC. Effects of azithromycin on gene expression profiles of Proinflammatory and anti-inflammatory mediators in the eyelid margin and conjunctiva of patients with Meibomian gland disease. JAMA Ophthalmol. 2015;133(10):1117–23.

50. Van Zuuren EJ, Fedorowicz Z. Interventions for rosacea. J Am Med Assoc. 2015;314(22):2403–4.

51. Donnenfeld E, Pflugfelder SC. MAJOR REVIEW topical ophthalmic cyclosporine: pharmacology and clinical uses. Surv Ophthalmol [Internet]. 2009;54(3):321–38. Available from:. https://doi.org/10.1016/j.survophthal.2009.02.002.

52. Sakassegawa-naves FE, Maria H, Ricci M, Kaplan B. Tacrolimus ointment for refractory posterior blepharitis. Curr Eye Res. 2017;42(11):1440–4.

Local and Systemic Associations

Vincent Michael Imbrogno

Dermatomyositis

Dermatomyositis refers to an autoimmune disease characterized primarily of skin and muscular involvement. The incidence is about 9 per one million with females affected about twice as commonly as males [1]. Average age of onset tends to be approximately 55 years of age [2]. A separately defined entity, juvenile dermatomyositis, is defined as having an earlier onset, from 5 to 14 years of age [3]. Yet another entity, amyopathic dermatomyositis, occurs with only skin manifestations and not the characteristic muscular findings [4]. There are 5 diagnostic criteria for the disease, with each positive criterion increasing the chance of diagnosis [5]. However, the necessary criteria for even suspected disease are eruptive dermatitis lesions typical of the disease. These lesions start as macular erythema distributed symmetrically over the body, typically in the posterior neck and shoulder areas (shawl sign) [2].

Nodules on the interphalangeal joint (Grotton's nodules) are also common [6]. The characteristic eyelid finding is the so-called heliotrope rash, which is a violaceous-hued erythema and edema of the upper, and occasionally lower, eyelids [7]. Skin manifestations precede muscular findings in approximately 50% of patients [8]. Muscle involvement is typically described as by proximal muscle weakness. In the presence of the rash, questions regarding difficulty raising from a chair, combing one's own hair, or climbing a flight of stairs may elucidate a positive response [9]. Lung [10] or esophageal [11] involvement are less common but more serious manifestations. Rarely, additional eye findings such as conjunctival hyperemia or polyposis, nystagmus, iritis, or retinal findings may be seen [12]. As stated previously, the diagnosis lies in a constellation of findings, first and foremost the characteristic skin findings. Also included are the proximal muscle weakness, an EMG demonstrating myopathy, elevated muscle enzymes in the serum, and inflammatory myopathy confirmed on muscle biopsy. The histologic findings of the skin manifestations show perivenular lymphocytic infiltrates; however, this is indistinguishable from other dermatologic diseases such as lupus erythematosus [13]. Myositis-specific antibody assays are also helpful in the diagnosis [14].

V. M. Imbrogno (✉)
Contemporary Ophthalmology of Erie,
Erie, PA, USA

© Springer Nature Switzerland AG 2021
A. V. Farooq, J. J. Reidy (eds.), *Blepharitis*, Essentials in Ophthalmology,
https://doi.org/10.1007/978-3-030-65040-7_3

Overlap syndromes with other rheumatologic diseases have been reported, with associated criteria needing to be met for those individual diseases [9]. An association between dermatomyositis and malignancies exist, and screening bloodwork and examination must be performed, as malignancies may present concurrently with the disease or even precede it [15]. Therapy targeting the skin findings include topical steroids, as the lesions can be quite pruritic. Also, patients tend to be photosensitive, and thus UV protection in the form of clothing or sunscreen is strongly advised. Muscular involvement is usually treated with oral steroids and a steroid-sparing agent, such as methotrexate or rituximab [16]. Close follow-up and communication with rheumatology and dermatology are recommended.

Systemic Lupus Erythematosus

Systemic lupus erythematosus (SLE) is a chronic autoimmune disease affecting nearly any or all organ systems. It typically follows a course of relapses and remissions, sometimes with relapses occurring in different organ systems or at different severities, making diagnosis difficult. Therefore, a clinician should always be considering this entity as a diagnosis when inflammatory conditions are observed on the eyelids [17]. Epidemiologically, the disease occurs in approximately 4–200 per 100,000 persons [18]. Women are affected more than men by a ratio of 9:1, with women of African American and Asian descent being more commonly affected than those of European ancestry. The age of onset is typically between 15 and 45 years of age [19].

The pathogenesis of SLE is not known, and is likely a combination of genetic predisposition and an inciting event such as an infection. B cell hyperactivity is a hallmark of the disease [20]. This in turn leads to immune complex deposition and a classic Type III hypersensitivity reaction. Due to its ability to mimic other diseases and its protean manifestations, 4 of 11 clinical findings must be present in order to diagnose a patient with definitive SLE. They include constitutional findings such as fever, malaise, myalgias, and weight loss or anorexia. Other important findings are photosensitivity, serositis, non-deforming migratory arthritis, kidney disease, and anemia [19]. Bloodwork will almost always show positivity to antinuclear antibodies; however, this alone is of limited benefit as nearly 33% of non-lupus patients may have positive ANA titers [21]. More specific antinuclear antibodies are anti-double-stranded DNA and anti-Smith antibodies. There is also an association with anti-SS-A and SS-B antibodies, but these are more closely associated with Sjögren's syndrome [17].

On ophthalmic and external examination, one of the most common findings is a malar rash, which is either a flat or slightly raised erythematous area over the malar prominences and nose. Another common finding is a discoid rash, which appears as a raised papular rash with keratotic scaling. On the eyelid, this may appear similar to chronic anterior blepharitis, with erythematous, thickened skin and madarosis. Other ocular manifestations range from anterior to posterior and include episcleritis and scleritis, sicca (with SLE often accompanying a diagnosis of Sjögren's syndrome), and cotton wool spots in the retina [19]. The retinal findings are consistent with the microvascular disease characteristic of SLE. Early clinical diagnosis is paramount to successful treatment, and therefore a careful review of systems and appropriate bloodwork should be considered in any patient with recurrent scleritis or blepharitis refractory to conservative treatment. Systemic therapy is indicated once the diagnosis is made, and typically consists of an initial corticosteroid followed most commonly by hydroxychloroquine [22]. In cases of severe or aggressive disease, most concerningly renal or CNS involvement, cyclophosphamide may be considered [23]. Biologics, including more recently belimumab, are becoming of increasing importance in long-term therapy [24].

Scleroderma

Another rheumatological disorder, scleroderma, involves extensive fibrosis of connective tissue. While the skin is usually involved, when the condition also involves visceral organs, it is referred to as progressive systemic sclerosis (PSS). Women are more frequently affected than men, with reported ratios as high as 9:1. Onset is generally in the childbearing years. One of the rarer diseases, the incidence has been reported to be 3–22 per million [25]. The underlying pathogenesis is a dysregulation of the capillaries and small blood vessels of the affected skin or organs. Initially, there is increased permeability causing edema. This is followed by a cascade of events resulting in fibroblast and myo-fibroblast activation, causing fibrosis of the surrounding tissue. Additionally, upregulation of platelet aggregation and inflammatory markers causes narrowing of the vessels, leading ultimately to ischemia [26]. Biomarkers can show positivity for antinuclear antibodies, anti-Scl70, and anti-RNA polymerase [27]. However, the diagnosis is usually made clinically from major and minor criteria established by the American College of Rheumatology [28].

Variants of the disease include CREST syndrome, an acronym standing for calcinosis, Raynaud's phenomenon, esophageal dysmotility, sclerodactyly, and telangiectasias. Clinically, the first sign noted on history is typically Raynaud's phenomenon, which happens in approximately 90% of patients [29]. The skin manifestations normally start in the extremities, moving centripetally to involve the upper arms and face. The skin change reflects the histologic findings, with initial edema followed by skin tightening and thickening. This, in turn, leads to loss of mobility and contracture. Ischemic disease can lead to infarcts and ulceration of the digits. Phenotypic variants include linear scleroderma, which can occur at a younger age. On the face, a lesion known as *coup de sabre* (sword stroke) can occur, which is frequently along the vertical midline. If the lesion develops early, this can result in facial asymmetry. The morphea variant involves only an isolated patch of skin, which results in characteristic indurated lesions. These typically undergo hyperpigmentation or can resolve over time.

Eye manifestations are representative of the global disease, causing an initial bout of edema followed by contracture of the skin. This can result in a woody or masked face appearance. For the eyelids, this results in decreased upper lid excursion, and blepharophimosis. If the disease extends to the lid margins, fibrosis of the dermal appendages may result in lash loss. Resultant corneal exposure is frequently a sequela of the condition. Other ocular findings are mostly a result of the associated microvascular disease. Iris atrophy, transillumination defects, and choroidal or retinal ischemia may develop [26].

Unfortunately, there are currently no available treatments that have been successful at treating the underlying disease. Management is therefore directed at supportive therapy of the involved systems. Oral steroids, generally considered a mainstay of controlling rheumatologic diseases, are generally avoided in scleroderma as this can worsen a patient's renal crisis [30]. Methotrexate, mycophenolate mofetil, and cyclophosphamide have all been used in an attempt to control the disease from a dermatologic standpoint [31]. For the eyes, controlling exposure keratopathy is of paramount importance. Long-term survival of the patient is most closely related to the extent of visceral involvement, with renal or lung involvement portending the worst prognosis [32].

Sjögren's Syndrome

Sjögren's syndrome (SS) is the autoimmune disease most frequently encountered by the ophthalmologist. As keratoconjunctivitis sicca is one of the primary symptoms, ophthalmology is frequently called upon early in the disease process for confirmation of diagnosis and management. Here, we will focus on the external aspects of SS and defer to resources outlining corneal diseases to better discuss the ocular surface disease manifestations. The prevalence of SS is about 10 in 10,000. Women of child-bearing age are the most commonly affected [33].

As with other autoimmune disorders, many patients have overlapping diseases. SS may be secondary to them, namely, rheumatoid arthritis, SLE, mixed connective tissue disease, and others [34]. A careful review of symptoms of a patient in whom SS is suspected is therefore warranted. Immunologically, a T-cell-mediated autoimmune response leads to gradual destruction of the exocrine glands, including the lacrimal and salivary glands; however, other mucous membranes including the trachea and vagina, may be affected. Microscopically, lymphocytic infiltration of the glands is seen, followed by destruction of the glandular structure [35]. Over time, fibrosis replaces the organizational structure of the gland [36].

Dermatologically, the skin tends to be dry (xeroderma), and is found in approximately two-thirds of patients [37]. Annular erythema is a rare finding in SS and can be found anywhere on the body but most commonly on the face. It consists of round lesions with an elevated erythematous border and pale center, similar to dermatophytosis [38]. A cutaneous vasculitis is also rarely seen, but is a harbinger of more severe systemic disease, as there is immune complex deposition in the small blood vessels [39]. The eyelids may show signs of dermatitis, with erythema and scaling similar to contact dermatitis or the heliotrope rash found in dermatomyositis [40].

Diagnostic workup begins with a focused history and physical, and includes questionnaires rating dry eye and dry mouth symptoms. Biopsy of the minor salivary gland can be performed for suspected cases, and it is still considered the gold standard for diagnosis [41]. Blood markers include ANA, which is present in 90% of cases but is fairly nonspecific. SS-A and SS-B antibodies are present in approximately 80–90% of the cases and are much more specific [42]. Treatment consists mostly of local therapy. Xeroderma and eyelid dermatitis are typically treated with skin moisturizers and cool, infrequent showers. Smoking and alcohol avoidance are strongly recommended. Treatment of the ocular surface is of utmost importance, beginning with lubricating agents. Cyclosporine, punctal occlusion, and autologous serum eyedrops are all advocated as therapy to avoid epithelial breakdown, melt, or infectious keratitis. Systemic immunosuppression may be considered.

Sarcoidosis

A multisystem inflammatory disease with myriad presentations, sarcoidosis is frequently referred to as "the great mimicker," especially when considering its dermatologic manifestations. The literature is focused most heavily on the pulmonary aspect of the disease, as this generally presents the gravest consequences to the patient. However, nearly any organ can become affected, including the skin, uveal tract, brain, liver, spleen, lymphatic system, GI tract, joints, or bones [43]. The incidence has been reported to be approximately 3–18 individuals per 100,000. Women are affected at approximately twice the rate of men, with the average age of diagnosis being approximately 50. African Americans are affected at a rate of double compared to whites, and 6 times more commonly than Asians or Hispanics [44].

Due to its protean manifestations, the initial presentation can vary widely. Löfgren's syndrome is a classic acute presentation, consisting of the triad of fever, eruptions of painful erythema nodosum, and ankle swelling. Hilar lymphadenopathy is frequently seen in conjunction with this [45]. Pulmonary symptoms are vague and consist most often of dyspnea and cough. The most frequent lung finding on imaging is hilar lymphadenopathy [46]. A staging system for lung involvement involves the presence of lymphadenopathy with or without parenchymal disease. Fibrotic parenchymal disease represents the final stage of sarcoidosis, and it is associated with pulmonary hypertension and right-sided heart failure [47].

A multitude of ocular presentations may occur. Anterior, intermediate, and posterior uveitis are all possibilities. Optic neuritis is an uncommon but concerning manifestation. Vasculopathy in the form of phlebitis with classic "candle wax drippings" may occur in the retina. Nodules on either the iris or conjunctiva can also be seen [48]. Lacrimal gland involvement can be seen in nearly 25% of sarcoid patients, and they may develop associated dry eye syndrome [49].

Dermatologically, sarcoid changes can be nonspecific. An entity that is exclusive to sarcoid is the misnomer "lupus pernio." It occurs on the face as indurated, violaceous lesions that tend to scar and cause disfigurement. They have the potential to erode into the bone, particularly into the nose and sinuses [50]. Worrisomely, lupus pernio is usually associated with severe pulmonary disease [51]. Often, however, the skin findings are not pathognomonic. Painful erythema nodosum, which are elevated, shiny nodules, can be seen throughout the body, usually on the extensor surfaces of the legs [52]. However, these lesions can also be seen in infectious or allergic diseases [53]. The skin findings may be even less specific. A case series of periocular sarcoid described cases of erythematous edema of the upper eyelid, upper lid dermatitis, a nodular lesion mimicking basal cell carcinoma, and bilateral medial canthal swelling. All were biopsy proven to be sarcoidosis [54]. Curiously, if the adnexal tissue is affected in a patient, they rarely have concomitant intraocular disease [55].

Given the nonspecific nature of the disease, biopsy of skin is frequently needed, and invariably will show noncaseating granulomas, which are pathognomonic. There may be associated multinucleated giant cells, which are usually surrounded by a cuff of lymphocytes [53]. Serum ACE and lysozyme are usually elevated, and should be a part of the workup in a patient with suspected sarcoid in the setting of concerning skin findings or uveitis. Treatment generally depends on the systems involved. For lung and cardiac disease, high-dose steroid therapy is generally initiated, followed by a steroid-sparing agent, such as methotrexate. Infliximab has been shown to be a promising steroid-sparing agent in the setting of lupus pernio. Topical corticosteroids are the mainstay of treatment for local symptoms, namely, eyedrops for uveitic manifestations, and ointment or cream for skin findings [56].

Rosacea

Rosacea is a chronic inflammatory disorder of the skin characterized by its tendency to affect the nose and malar eminences of the face. It is a common condition, with some studies reporting as high as 10% of the population being affected [57]. Women are more commonly affected than men, although men are more likely to suffer from the phymatous subtype, which manifests as skin thickening and rhinophyma. Diagnosis is usually made after the age of 30 [58]. Fair-skinned patients of European descent are most commonly affected.

While there are four main subtypes of phenotypic manifestations, there is significant overlap in any given patient, with age of onset, degree of inflammation, and duration of disease all important aspects of clinical findings. Erythematotelangiectatic (ETR) disease is characterized by episodes of flushing and persistent erythema of the face, frequently accompanied by telangiectasias. Papulopustular disease involves transient papules or pustules in the same distribution as ETR disease. Phymatous findings are associated with nodular skin thickening, most commonly on the nose and cheeks [59]. Extreme rhinophyma can result from chronic untreated disease. Ocular rosacea involves the eyelids and conjunctiva. Eyelid disease mainly consists of posterior blepharitis and telangiectasia. The meibomian gland orifices are often distorted or obliterated, resulting in frequent chalazia or hordeola.

Long-term ocular rosacea results in meibomian gland deficiency and dry eye disease. The inferior conjunctiva is most commonly involved, with injection and chemosis. Mechanical irritation of the inferior cornea can occur, resulting in inferior keratitis, epithelial breakdown, sterile ulceration, or corneal neovascularization [60]. Infestation with the skin mite Demodex may either be a comorbidity, or a triggering cause of the disease, as chitin from the mite's exoskeleton has been shown to activate toll-like receptor 2, an important signal in the inflammatory pathway [61]. Matrix metalloproteinase-9 is also expressed at higher levels on rosacea patients, indicating a dysregulation of inflammation [62]. Coagulase-negative *S. aureus* and *H. pylori* have also been proposed as contributors to the pathogenesis of rosacea [63, 64].

The diagnosis of rosacea is almost always made clinically. Histological findings are nonspecific, and so biopsy is rarely indicated. Therapy is directed at controlling local disease. Environmental triggers should be avoided if possible. These include alcohol intake, smoking, spicy food, exposure to extreme temperatures, exercise and physical or psychological stress [65]. Barrier skin moisturizers are a mainstay of initial therapy. UV-blocking sunscreen should always be applied prior to sun exposure. FDA-approved topical medications include sodium sulfacetamide, brimonidine, azelaic acid, and metronidazole. Topical ivermectin cream has shown to be effective at controlling the disease. Its effects are likely due to anti-parasitic activity against *Demodex* species as well as anti-inflammatory properties. Tetracyclines remain the gold standard for systemic therapy. Doxycycline, 40-200 mg daily, has been shown to reduce symptoms in patients with rosacea. Doxycycline is capable of both decreasing the expression of matrix metalloproteinase and inhibiting neutrophil function. Therefore, tetracyclines are used for their anti-inflammatory effects more so than for their antibacterial properties [66]. With timely and adequate treatment, patients with rosacea fare well, although they should be informed of the chronic and fluctuating nature of their disease.

Seborrhea

Seborrhea, or seborrheic dermatitis, is a chronic inflammatory skin condition, usually affecting the face, scalp, axilla, groin, and back. Included in the spectrum of disease is dandruff, a much more common condition affecting nearly 50% of the adult population [67]. Seborrhea, although less common, still affects about 1–3% of the total population [68]. It presents in a trimodal manner, with one peak being in the first year of life. When present on the scalp, this is most commonly referred to as "cradle cap," with infants also being affected in the facial and diaper areas. The second peak is during puberty and early adulthood. Finally, a third peak occurs from 40 to 60, with similar manifestations to those seen in the adolescent cohort [69]. Men are more commonly affected than women, with exacerbations being brought about by cold temperatures, low humidity, or periods of stress [70].

Interestingly, a disproportionately large percentage of patients suffering from seborrhea have an immunocompromised status. Organ-transplant, lymphoma, or HIV-positive patients have all been shown to have an increased risk for the disease [71]. In particular, approximately 50% of HIV-positive patients suffer from seborrhea [72]. Furthermore, patients suffering from neurologic diseases such as Parkinson's, tardive dyskinesia, or traumatic brain injury, all have higher rates of seborrhea compared to the general population [69]. The pathophysiology of seborrhea is poorly understood, but with the knowledge of the increased prevalence in immunocompromised and neurologic patients, it can be assumed that both immune status and neuroendocrine dysfunction have a role to play.

A common commensal yeast, *Malassezia*, has been studied as a potential culprit. While *Malassezia* has been isolated from the majority of patients with normal skin, it has been shown in seborrhea patients to be able to penetrate into the stratum corneum of the skin, releasing free fatty acids, an environment that allows the yeast to thrive. This cascade causes breakdown of the epidermal water barrier, contributing to water loss [73]. The yeast's ability to act pathogenically in seborrhea patients is not clearly understood. Clinically, the hallmark of the disease is patches of scaly, greasy-appearing erythema with flaky skin. It is frequently accompanied by pruritis, which is especially true of scalp involvement [74].

The eyelid findings are an extension of the general disease, and typically presents as an anterior blepharitis, with crusting or scaling on the lid lashes with skin debris. The posterior lid may also become involved, and consist of meibomian gland dysfunction, leading to evaporative tear dysfunction and dry eye [75]. Treatment is directed at the area of involvement. Scalp involvement can be successfully managed with over-the-counter dandruff shampoos containing agents such as selenium sulfide, zinc pyrithione, or coal tar [76]. Given the likelihood of *Malassezia* overgrowth, topical antifungal agents such as ketoconazole have been advocated [77]. Skin disease of the face, back, or other body areas includes topical antifungals or calcineurin inhibitors such as tacrolimus [78]. Skin hygiene, including gentle exfoliation of the scaly patches and judicious use of topical steroids, remains a mainstay of therapy. For the eyelids, warm compresses aid in expressing turbid meibomian secretions. Baby shampoo lid scrubs are effective at clearing skin debris from the lash base and meibomian orifice. Rarely, the associated inflammation from the disease necessitates a short-term course of topical steroids or systemic antibiotics, such as doxycycline [75].

Atopic Dermatitis

Atopic dermatitis represents an IgE-mediated-hypersensitivity, usually to external allergens or triggers. It is frequently associated with other atopic diseases, including food allergies, allergic rhinitis, and allergic asthma [79]. The prevalence of the disease is increasing, with nearly 15–20% of children and 1–3% of adults being affected [80]. This represents a nearly tripling of disease burden over the last 40–50 years. Diagnosis is typically made before age 5, with most cases diagnosed before 6 months [81]. The majority of adult cases represent a continuation of the disease since childhood. Less than 20% of patients are diagnosed with atopic dermatitis after adolescence [82]. There is relative parity amongst the sexes, with males being affected at a slightly higher rate than females. Typically, however, males tend to have more persistent and severe disease [83].

Although common, the exact underlying pathogenesis of atopic dermatitis is not well understood. Recently, interest in the filaggrin gene has been demonstrating the importance of skin barrier dysfunction as a pathway toward disease. Filaggrin is an important protein for epidermal differentiation, and recent studies have shown downregulation of filaggrin can cause skin barrier dysfunction. This may allow allergens to penetrate deeper into the epidermis, increasing the likelihood of contact with mast cells and thus triggering an allergic response. It is unknown however, whether internalization of an allergen causes downregulation of filaggrin, or if the reverse is true [84]. Only about 30% of atopic patients present with a true filaggrin mutation, suggesting that the etiology is at least partly environmental [85]. Diagnosis is usually made by history and physical examination. While there has been an extensive classification criteria established, clinically this can be unwieldy. Nonetheless, pruritis is a hallmark of the disease, and a necessary criterion for diagnosis [86].

The physical findings vary, mostly according to patient age and duration of disease. In infants and young children, the most common areas affected are the antecubital and popliteal fossae. The lesions present as eczema: erythematous areas of weeping pustules that crust over. In more advanced cases, these pustules will coalesce into open areas of weeping skin, which are prone to secondary infection. The disease then spreads to involve other areas of the body, namely the cheeks, chin, and forehead. Importantly, the diaper area and nose are almost never affected, and their involvement during an evaluation should strongly suggest an alternate diagnosis. The child is frequently seen rubbing at the areas, suggesting pruritis. Elsewhere on the skin, non-eczematous areas are generally xerotic, showing flaky or cracked skin.

As the child ages, the lesions can become chronic, and skin thickening may develop over the affected areas due to repeated and excessive rubbing [87]. Into adulthood, the areas take on an erythematous appearance, with thin, dry, and scaly skin [88]. Skin folds tend to be increased or pronounced. The eyelids and facial skin are representative of this change. In adults, frequently the skin becomes taut, and subsequent cicatricial ectropion can occur. The anterior lid margin can become involved with flaking of the skin resulting in increased lid scurf [89]. Ocular involvement usually presents in the form of atopic conjunctivitis. There are fine papillae on the tarsal conjunctiva. Subepithelial fibrosis may ensue in poorly controlled or aggressive cases. Posterior capsular or anterior shield-shaped lens opacities have been reported [88].

Topical therapy remains the first-line treatment. Barrier moisturizers, topical steroids, and steroid-sparing agents such as tacrolimus are all considered primary tools in achieving stability of the disease. Typically, when remission is achieved, patients are well advised to continue moisturization, and occasionally consider weekly application of topical steroids to avoid relapses [90]. Regimens are individually based, depending on response to therapy and side-effect profiles [91]. Topical long-term high-dose steroid therapy is associated with skin thinning, an important consideration for the ophthalmologist considering the already thinner skin of the lids. In children, recalcitrant disease despite therapy should warrant consideration for food allergies. Consultation with a pediatric allergist is likely warranted [92]. For systemic therapies, immunomodulators are considered. Cyclosporine, methotrexate, azathioprine, and mycophenolate mofetil are all advocated as being effective at controlling disease [93]. Currently, the biologic agent dupilumab is the only FDA-approved biologic to combat atopic dermatitis, with a litany of additional agents being actively investigated [94]. If systemic disease is present, or systemic therapy warranted, coordination with dermatologic, rheumatologic, or allergic specialists is advised.

Ichthyosis

Ichthyosis is an umbrella term for a spectrum of dermatologic diseases, all characterized by hyperkeratosis and scaling. A majority of these diseases are congenital and inherited in a Mendelian fashion. There have been more than 30 alleles identified as having mutations resulting in ichthyosis [95]. Pathologically, all congenital forms of ichthyosis involve abnormal development of the two outermost layers of the epithelium: the stratum granulosum and stratum corneum [96]. In ichthyosis, hyperproliferation, inappropriate aggregation, or delayed shedding of cells lead to an accumulation of skin, resulting in macroscopic phenotypic findings, which vary due to the underlying genetic defect unique to each entity [95]. In addition to the congenital entities, ichthyosis can be a clinical finding in larger syndromic diseases, or secondary to other disease processes. The plethora of individual diseases, underlying genetic characteristics, clinical findings, or primary causes in the cases of secondary disease are beyond the scope of this chapter. This section will therefore focus on those most commonly associated with the eye in general, and the lids in particular.

Ichthyosis vulgaris (IV) is the most common genetic variant, affecting approximately 1 in 300 individuals [97]. Findings of the disease present within the first year of life, uniformly demonstrating hyperkeratosis of the soles and palms. The torso and extensor surfaces are commonly affected [98]. Eyelid involvement is typically manifested as scaling of the eyelids and lashes. Congenital ichthyosiform erythroderma (CIE) is an autosomal recessive disease that is much less common. Patients suffering from CIE frequently present at birth as "collodion" babies, referring to the tight membrane surrounding the infant following delivery. Eyelids of CIE patients are similar to those with IV, with the scales being finer and whiter [97]. Additionally, they may have madarosis, posterior blepharitis, and upper lid ectropion [99].

Lamellar ichthyosis is another autosomal recessive variant, with possibly the most significant eyelid findings. In addition to being collodion babies, there is dramatic shortening of the anterior lamellae with resultant ectropion of both the upper and lower lids. Additionally, there is significant meibomian gland dysfunction and dropout [100]. The conjunctival and corneal disease of these patients is a direct extension of exposure and evaporative tear dysfunction, resulting in keratitis, melt, perforation, or vascularization. Epidermolytic hyperkeratosis is autosomal dominant, with highlighting features including more erythematous lesions with skin fragility and blistering. Due to frequent breakdown of the skin of these patients, secondary bacterial infections are of increased concern. The disease tends to decrease in severity with age [97].

In all cases, the diagnosis is frequently made due to the overt skin changes, with subsequent genetic testing revealing the underlying defect. Other non-skin system involvement would point an ophthalmologist in the direction of one of the many syndromes that include ichthyosis (KID, Sjogren-Larsson, IAFP, Refsum, etc.). Presentation is usually at or shortly after birth; therefore, any patient presenting at a later age should strongly suggest either mild or acquired disease [101].

Treatment of the eye is typically directed toward lid disease and protection of the ocular surface. Prophylactic lubrication, even in the absence of active corneal disease, is paramount given the high risk of future breakdown. Frequent preservative-free tears or ophthalmic ointment should be advocated. Moisture chambers, especially while sleeping, should be considered for any patient with significant ectropion, poor Bell's, or incomplete lid blink [102]. Therapy directed at the lids consists of moisturization and mechanical desquamation. Gentle lid massage can both relax the anterior lamellae and manually debride excess skin, thus allowing the lids to conform to a more normal contour [103]. Five or 10% N-acetylcysteine can be used topically, as it has anti-proliferative effects and likely leads to decreased epithelium formation. Studies have demonstrated excellent efficacy and even resolution of ectropion with its use, often in conjunction with the keratolytic 5% urea cream [104].

Surgical interventions are commonly deployed to alleviate disease burden. Hyaluronic acid filler can be considered a less invasive option than skin grafting; however, it is generally considered a temporizing measure until a more definitive procedure is done [105]. As with any surgical correction of cicatricial ectropion, the goal is to improve lid functionality and protection of the globe. Autologous skin grafts remain the most common surgical approach, with mucous membrane and transposition flaps also being reported [99].

Graft-Versus-Host Disease

In the modern era, bone marrow or peripheral blood transplantation has become an invaluable tool in the treatment of hematologic malignancies or disorders. Broadly defined as autologous (the patient receiving his/her own cells) or allogenic (from a matched donor), cells are harvested from either the bone marrow, peripheral blood, or umbilical cord. However, colloquially, the term bone marrow transplant (BMT) has evolved to encompass all of these techniques. These cells are then transplanted into the recipient patient, usually after they have undergone a regimen to remove all native blood cells (conditioning) [106].

Graft-versus-host disease therefore represents an immune response whereby the transplanted cells attack the recipient tissue. It occurs with allogenic transplantation. A series of risk factors exist that increase the chances of GVHD, including female donor cells transplanted into male recipients or advanced age of the recipient [107]. Additionally, patients who receive peripheral blood transplants tend to have a higher risk of GVHD when compared to bone marrow recipients [108]. There is anywhere from a 10–90% prevalence for developing ocular GVHD [109]. Such a large range is likely due to several factors, such as inclusion criteria, duration of observation, and newer pre-BMT treatment modalities, which decrease the risk of GVHD. Nevertheless, this disease represents a significant morbidity of BMT.

Classically, GVHD has been described as being acute or chronic. Acute GVHD is defined as occurring within the first 100 days after BMT, and chronic occurring after the first 100 [110]. This timeline is arbitrary, however, and a more accurate delineation can be explained histopathologically. Acute GVHD involves infiltration of T cells into the tissue of the skin, GI tract and liver, causing necrosis and in the case of the GI tract, biliary obstruction [111]. Rarely lung or vascular involvement can occur [109].

Acute ocular GVDH involves infiltration of the lacrimal gland, causing "stasis" of tears due to obliteration of the lumen of the gland, resulting in severe aqueous tear deficiency [112]. The skin of the face and eyelid may become involved, with varying degrees of severity. Typically, a morbilliform maculopapular rash or erythroderma may occur. Outright desquamation, clinically indistinguishable from toxic epidermal necrolysis, is a feared outcome [113]. Desquamating eyelids may evolve into cicatricial ectropion. The meibomian glands can become hyperemic, with gland dropout and accompanying evaporative tear dysfunction [114]. Conjunctival manifestations of acute ocular GVDH exhibit hyperemia and chemosis, or outright epithelial sloughing with pseudomembanes and possible symblepharon formation. The eyelids may have resultant entropion. The cornea is usually affected secondarily by sicca due to loss of lacrimal gland function, but itself may suffer from epithelial sloughing leading to melt and perforation [110]. Posterior subcapsular cataracts can also be seen, but it is unclear if this represents GVHD, or is a side effect from systemic medications, particularly steroids [106].

Chronic GVHD is characterized by fibroblastic infiltration into the tissues, resulting in atrophy. The meibomian gland structures of the lids can become completely obliterated [115]. Of particular importance for chronic management, the lacrimal gland can become severely affected, and it is assumed that the injury is irreversible [116]. Chronic erythema and congestion of the lids can lead to nasolacrimal duct obstruction. While this may be generally thought of as helpful in the treatment of dry eye disease, obstructions can happen more distally, resulting in episodes of dacryocystitis [117]. Treatment of ocular GVHD is targeted primarily at protecting the ocular surface, through reducing inflammation and lubrication. While acute ocular GVDH is uncommon, it unfortunately carries with it a poor prognosis for survival [118].

For acute ocular and systemic GVHD, systemic steroids remain the treatment of choice. However, even with high-dose steroids, there is only a 50% response rate, and non-responders have a dismal 5-year prognosis [119]. Because the pathology of acute GVHD is so interlinked with T-cell activity, extracorporeal photophoresis has been advocated as rescue therapy for steroid resistant disease, or as adjuvant therapy [120]. For strictly acute ocular disease, systemic therapy is not warranted. In the event of conjunctival or corneal sloughing, protection with bandage contact lens has been advocated, but judicious use of antibiotics is necessary, as is close follow-up [121]. Amniotic membrane is a therapeutic option in the event of conjunctival or corneal epithelium loss. Self-retaining amniotic rings can be considered for corneal disease; however, if there is concern for symblepharon formation, suturing of amniotic membrane to the tarsal conjunctiva and placement of a symblepharon ring should be considered. This has demonstrated efficacy in the setting of Stevens-Johnson syndrome, which follows a similar course [122].

For acute and chronic ocular GVHD, intensive tear replacement therapy is warranted, including frequent application of preservative-free artificial tears and lubricating ointments. Punctal occlusion may be considered; concomitant punctal stenosis may make sizing of plugs difficult, at which point cautery may be an option. Topical cyclosporine A 0.05% BID should also be considered for its effect against T cells and general anti-inflammatory properties. However, unlike Sjogren's syndrome, it should not be anticipated to improve Schirmer's [106]. Autologous serum eyedrops at 20% concentration used four times daily has also been shown to be beneficial to GVHD patients for their anti-inflammatory properties [123]. Topical N-acetylcysteine can aid in the treatment of filamentary keratitis. Meibomian gland disease is treated with warm compresses, baby shampoo lid scrubs, fish or flax seed oil, and doxycycline for its ability to inhibit matrix metalloproteinase [124]. Scleral lenses have shown promise in providing comfort in severe cases, as they allow the surface continuous hydration and desiccation protection [125]. Entropion or ectropion repair is advised to further protect the ocular surface, provided the primary conjunctival or skin disease is well controlled.

Epidermolysis Bullosa

Epidermolysis bullosa (EB) is a related group of inherited disorders, all with a common underlying pathology of stress-induced blistering of the skin. Pathologically, there is impaired connectivity of skin cells, with characteristics unique to the depth of involvement. Epidermolysis bullosa simplex is caused by a defect in either keratin 5 [126] or 14 [127], and results in intraepidermal splitting. Junctional EB occurs at the level of the lamina lucida and is usually defective in laminins [128]. Dystrophic EB, inherited in either an autosomal dominant or recessive fashion, affects the area below the lamina densa, and usually represents a defect in Type VII collagen [129]. While their underlying genetic abnormalities and specific phenotypic expressions are beyond the scope of this chapter, those affecting the eyelid and eye surface are worthy of attention. EB simplex almost never involves the eye or surrounding tissues and tends to have the mildest course of all EB variants. A particular subtype of EB simplex called Dowling-Meara syndrome can involve the eye, with conjunctival bullae and eyelid inflammation being typical [130].

Junctional EB has the potential to develop blisters in the periocular area, leading to cicatricial ectropion and corneal exposure, with its accompanying complications. Furthermore, recurrent corneal erosions and associated scarring may occur [131]. Dystrophic EB is further divided into autosomal dominant vs. recessive. Dominant disease rarely, if ever, involves the eye, whereas recessive dystrophic EB has the most severe ocular manifestations. Cicatricial ectropion, recurrent erosions, limbal stem cell deficiency, symblepharon, and corneal neovascularization have all been reported [132].

Diagnosis is typically made using a combination of skin biopsy and genetic testing. A blister is elicited by rolling a pencil eraser over the patient's skin to develop a fresh blister. A biopsy is then taken and using electron microscopy, the level of separation can be visualized. Furthermore, immunofluorescence can aid in determining the level of involvement, and demonstrate the absence of certain adherence molecules [130]. Genetic testing will help reveal the underlying abnormality, but at present there are no successful gene replacement therapies available.

Treatment at this point remains supportive. For corneal erosions, frequent application of preservative-free tears and nighttime ointment should be encouraged. Due to the underlying genetics, corneal resurfacing procedures are generally ineffective, and long-term bandage contact lens wear may provide more symptomatic relief for the patient. Close follow-up is warranted in these cases to avoid contact lens–associated bacterial infections. Symblepharon formation can be treated similarly to other etiologies, with lysis of the adhesions and forniceal reconstruction either by mucosal grafting or by amniotic membrane transplantation [132]. Patients with limbal stem cell deficiency are potential candidates for either transplantation or keratoprosthesis. Cicatricial ectropion can be repaired with skin grafting, although wound healing is difficult in these patients, and so reoperations are common.

Pemphigus

Pemphigus is a group of related autoimmune diseases, all with the clinical manifestations of blistering of the skin and mucous membranes. The majority of cases have an underlying genetic predisposition; however, associations with neoplastic diseases and certain drug use have been well documented. All are characterized by IgG autoantibodies directed against proteins responsible for intercellular adherence, namely, desmoglein [133]. Pemphigus vulgaris (PV) is the most common of these diseases, representing about 70% of all pemphigus cases [134]. Age of onset is between 40 and 60 years of age, with parity between the sexes and races [135]. Typically, PV presents with oral mucosal lesions that blister, denude, and are prone to secondary infection. The disease then spreads to include the skin, particularly the face, scalp, upper extremities, and groin [136]. The lesions appear as thin-walled bullae, which are easily ruptured. Lateral extension of the bullae with pressure is characteristic (Nikolsky's sign). The ruptured bullae then heal slowly. Pemphigus foliaceus presents in a similar fashion; however, the blisters are more superficial and therefore break easily.

Exfoliative findings on the skin are more prominent, and the mucous membranes are rarely involved [137]. Paraneoplastic pemphigus is usually associated with hematologic neoplasms, particularly non-Hodgkin lymphoma or chronic lymphocytic leukemia. However, solid organ tumors including colon, pancreatic, lung, breast, and others have been reported [138]. The mucous membrane involvement in paraneoplastic pemphigus tends to be the most severe, with up to 70% of patients having conjunctival disease [139]. Drug-induced pemphigus is caused by an ever-expanding list of medications. The classic example is penicillamine. Drugs containing either a thiol or phenol moiety are the most likely culprits. The disease is usually limited to the skin, and is preceded by annular erythema or urticarial rash, followed by more classic lesions [140]. Histologically, immunofluorescence demonstrates IgG deposition in the intercellular space in all patients.

For PV, the area of involvement is just above the basal epithelial cells. Separation of the skin in pemphigus foliaceus is intraepidermal, explaining the clinical finding of more superficial blisters [141]. Eyelid involvement can result in lid notching, trichiasis, and cicatricial ectropion. Lesions affecting the lid margin can cause blepharitis [142]. Pemphigoid foliaceus may have extensive scaling and lid margin keratinization [143]. The conjunctiva, when involved, can range from refractory conjunctivitis to epithelial sloughing and cicatricial disease. The cornea is usually only secondarily affected due to exposure or tear film instability. The mainstay of therapy is systemic steroids accompanied by a steroid-sparing agent, usually azathioprine. However, mycophenolate mofetil or cyclophosphamide can be considered in patients intolerant of azathioprine [133]. For severe disease, IVIG can be implemented [144]. Rituximab, the anti-CD20 inhibitor, has shown promise as an alternate therapy [145].

Acute conjunctival involvement requires debridement of necrotic tissue and if necessary, placement of a symblepharon ring to present cicatrization [146]. In the case of foliaceus, lid scrubs and warm compresses can help delay keratinization of the lid margin. Frequent use of artificial tears and lubricants can aid in protecting the cornea from exposure. Correction of trichiasis includes epilation, either manual (temporary) or via cryotherapy or electrolysis (permanent) [147]. Any correction to lid shortening from the disease should only be performed during quiescence, rather than risk reactivation of the disease [148]. With the advent of high-dose steroid and anti-inflammatory therapy, mortality from pemphigus has dropped from 90% to 10% [133].

Pyoderma Gangrenosum

Pyoderma gangrenosum is a rare autoimmune disease typified by ulcerating lesions. The classic lesion is a pustule that ulcerates centrally and extends peripherally with a violaceous border. Other appearances including ulcerative, bullous, or vegetative have been described [149]. The etiology is not well understood, but appears to be dysregulation of the immune system. Poor trafficking of neutrophils and aberrant T-cell function have been postulated as potential underlying culprits [150]. Nevertheless, the lesions typically present at an area of trauma (pathergy) including surgical wounds [151]. The disease affects approximately 10 people per million. Women are affected at a slightly higher rate than men, with the age range reported between 20 and 50 [152]. Associated systemic diseases include inflammatory bowel disease, myeloproliferative disorders, and rheumatoid arthritis [153]. Histopathologic findings are somewhat nonspecific. Neutrophil infiltration is the most consistent finding, with necrosis of the tissue and a chronic inflammatory infiltrate also commonly being observed. Clinical suspicion, therefore, must be very high in order to achieve a proper diagnosis.

Eyelid manifestations are similar to those elsewhere on the body. Although eyelid and ocular involvement are rare, the consequences are quite severe, and therefore rapid diagnosis is key, as therapy is effective at inducing remission. Case reports in the literature have demonstrated periocular skin disease, peripheral ulcerative keratitis, orbital involvement, and scleritis. Five case reports ended with loss of the eye, and another 9 were left with permanent visual deficits [154]. High-dose oral steroids are the first-line treatment, with a steroid-sparing agent either starting shortly after or concomitantly [155]. Azathioprine, dapsone, or oral cyclosporine are all possibilities. Surgical repair must if at all possible be delayed until after control of the disease, as this may exacerbate the ulcerative process. With treatment, the prognosis is quite good; however, the rate of recurrence after cessation of therapy have been reported to be as high as 40% [156].

Acrodermatitis Enteropathica

Acrodermatitis enteropathica is an autosomal recessive disorder characterized by poor absorption of zinc from the GI tract [157]. The initial manifestations occur at or shortly after birth. Scaly plaques, eczematous or vesicular lesions erupt on the digits, face and eyelids, or inguinal area [158]. Infants will also show failure to thrive, irritability, and increased susceptibility to fungal infections. Skin infections are of particular importance, due to the chronic open areas. Additionally, as zinc is an important cofactor for multiple enzymes, patients frequently present with an immunocompromised status [159]. The differential diagnosis in an infant with such facial lesions can be extensive, including congenital herpetic infection, epidermolysis bullosa, atopic dermatitis, or congenital celiac disease, among others [160]. Therapy includes zinc supplementation [161]. Dramatic improvement of the skin appearance is observed within the first 48 hours of oral therapy initiation [162].

Infectious Diseases

Certain infectious processes have specific eyelid findings. Some, such as Demodex infestation, are mild and typically limited to the face. Others, such as herpes zoster virus (HZV), can be severe and affect any location on the body. This section will briefly cover the most common infectious sources of lid disease, specifically their unique findings and treatment recommendations.

Demodicosis infestation can involve either the *Demodex folliculorum* or *Demodex brevis* organism. There is a gradient of infestation, as colonization with the mites is nearly universal by the age of 70 [163]. Therefore, pathology is likely related to over-infestation rather than their simple presence. *D. folliculorum* typically infests the lashes, causing an anterior blepharitis. The mite burrows into hair and lash follicles [164]. Its presence creates a characteristic cylindrical dandruff at the base of the lash, which is pathognomonic. *D. brevis* occupies the meibomian and sebaceous glands. Infestation with *D. brevis* causes a posterior blepharitis, with marginal erythema, keratinization, and recurrent chalazia [165]. Chronic infestation can cause conjunctivitis and inferior keratitis with pannus [166]. Demodex infestation has been proposed to be an underlying factor in rosacea [167]. Therapy consists of lid scrubs with baby shampoo to debride the lash collarettes. Fifty percent tea tree oil has been shown to be effective at controlling the disease; however, this can cause significant eye irritation [168]. Lower concentrations have been proven to be effective. Terpinen-4-ol has recently been demonstrated to be the most active ingredient in tea tree oil and is available as a prepared lid wipe (Cliradex) [169]. While independent investigations have demonstrated reduced Demodex counts with its use, it has yet to be FDA approved [170]. Topical and oral ivermectin have been shown to be effective for demodicosis of the facial skin.

Angular blepharitis is typically caused by the bacterium *Moraxella lucanata*. The lateral, or in some cases medial, canthus and eyelid are affected. The skin is erythematous, fissured, and scaly. There can be an associated conjunctivitis. Culturing is not necessary; however, viral infections such as HZV or herpes simplex virus (HSV) should be ruled out. Treatment involves lid scrubs and warm compresses. Additionally, topical antibiotic preparations such as erythromycin or bacitracin can be helpful. In the case of severe or refractory disease, oral tetracyclines, such as doxycycline hyclate, can be used [171].

HSV type 1 (and occasionally HSV type 2) can present as a blepharoconjunctivitis. It can occur either during the primary infection or at recurrences. A vesicular eruption occurs over the eyelid, usually confined to the periorbital tissue [172]. These vesicles then rupture and crust over, healing without scarring over 2–3 weeks. There can be an associated conjunctival papillary reaction. Corneal findings at the time of primary infection are usually mild and consist of punctate keratitis [173]. Secondary infections have a similar appearance on external exam, but there is increased likelihood of stromal or endothelial corneal disease. Other HSV ocular manifestations are protean, and include anterior uveitis, iris atrophy, vitritis, and acute retinal necrosis (ARN) [172]. Treatment for eyelid manifestations, especially in the presence of conjunctival or corneal disease, may include oral acyclovir 400 mg 5 times daily or oral valacyclovir 500 mg three times daily. Distortion of eyelid anatomy is rare; however, long-term risk for corneal disease should be of concern.

HZV can also present with a blepharoconjunctivitis; however, the findings are usually are more prominent [174]. Primary infection usually occurs during childhood as chickenpox (varicella). The virus then remains dormant in the trigeminal nerve ganglion. Reactivation can occur at any time later in life but is most common in the sixth decade. Episodes typically initiate as a prodrome of fever and malaise. Next, a maculopapular rash on an erythematous base occurs along the V1 dermatome [175]. The lesions rapidly progress to vesicles which rupture, crust, and form into eschar.

Pain is usually a prominent symptom, although in more elderly patients the lesions may be totally asymptomatic. As lesions heal, normal lid anatomy may become distorted, with trichiasis, ectropion, entropion, or punctal stenosis all possible. Corneal involvement is frequently seen, particularly with nasociliary branch involvement, which causes vesicle eruption on the tip of the nose (Hutchinson's sign) [174]. Corneal disease can vary from punctate keratitis to stromal infiltrates, geographic ulcers, melt, and perforation. Other intraocular findings include uveitis, sectoral iris atrophy, retinitis, or vasculitis [176]. Therapy consists of oral acyclovir 800 mg 5 times daily or oral valacyclovir 1 gram 3 times daily. Rapid initiation of antiviral therapy has been shown to reduce the risk of postherpetic neuralgia, which can be extremely debilitating and recalcitrant to pain therapy once established [177].

A summary of the common eyelid findings in systemic diseases is presented in Table 3.1.

Table 3.1 Common eyelid findings in systemic diseases

Disease	Findings
Autoimmune	
Dermatomyositis	Heliotrope rash
Systemic lupus erythematosus	Erythema, thickening, madarosis
Scleroderma	Tight, thickened skin; blepharophimosis
Sjögren's	Erythema, scaling
Sarcoidosis	Nodules, lupus pernio changes
Pemphigus	Bullae, lid notching, trichiasis
Pyoderma gangrenosum	Sterile ulceration with violaceous border
Dermatologic	
Rosacea	Telangiectasia, chalazia
Acrodermatitis enteropathica	Scales, eczema, vesicles
Epidermolysis bullosa	Blisters, cicatricial ectropion, symblepharon
Atopy	Erythematous, thickening, cicatricial ectropion
Seborrhea	Scale, greasy erythema
Ichthyosis	Thickened, scaly skin, cicatricial ectropion
Infectious	
Demodex	Lash collarettes
Angular blepharitis	Fissured erythema
Herpes simplex	Periorbital vesicular rash
Varicella zoster	V1 vesicular rash, eschar
Miscellaneous	
Graft-versus-host disease	Maculopapular rash, desquamating (rare), marginal keratinization

Compliance with Ethical Requirements

Conflict of Interest:
Vincent M. Imbrogno declares that he has no conflict of interest.

Informed Consent:
No human studies were carried out by the authors for this chapter.

Animal Studies:
No animal studies were carried out by the authors for this chapter.

References

1. Bendewald MJ, Wetter DA, Li X, Davis MD. Incidence of dermatomyositis and clinically amyopathic dermato-myositis: a population-based study in Olmsted County, Minnesota. Arch Dermatol. 2010;146(1):26–30. https://doi.org/10.1001/archdermatol.2009.328.
2. Marvi U, et al. Clinical presentation and evaluation of dermatomyositis. Indian J Dermatol. 2012;57(5):375–81. https://doi.org/10.4103/0019-5154.100486.
3. Paller AS. Juvenile dermatomyositis and overlap syndromes. Adv Dermatol. 1995;10:309–26.
4. Pearson CM. Polymyositis and dermatomyositis. In: McCarty DJ, editor. Arthritis. 9th ed. Philadelphia: Lea & Febiger; 1979. p. 748.
5. Bohan A, Peter JB. Polymyositis and dermatomyositis. N Engl J Med. 1975;292(part I):344–7.
6. Euwer RL, Sontheimer RD. Amyopathic dermatomyositis (dermatomyositis sine myositis). J Am Acad Dermaol. 1991;24:959–66.
7. Callen JP. Dermatomyositis. Dermatol Clin. 1983;1:461–73.

8. Rockerbie NR, Woo TY, Callen JP, et al. Cutaneous changes of dermatomyositis precede muscle weakness. J Am Acad Dermatol. 1989;20:629–32.
9. Kovacs SO, Kovacs SC. Dermatomyositis. J Am Acad Dermatol. 1998;39:899–920.
10. Tazelaar HD, Viggiano RW, Pickersgill J, et al. Interstitial lung disease in polymyositis and dermatomyositis. Am Rev Respir Dis. 1990;141:727.
11. Vitali C, Scuito M, Rossi B. Rectal incontinence due to an unusual localization of the myositic process in the external sphincter of a patient with dermatomyositis. Arthritis Rheum. 1991;34:1337.
12. Ibanez HE, Bardenstein DS, Korman NJ, et al. Exuberant conjunctival pseudopolyposis in a patient with dermato-myositis. Ann Ophthalmol. 1993;25:326–7.
13. Shetler D, Saornil M, et al. Pathology of the lids. In: Albert M, et al., editors. Albert & Jakobiec's principles and practice of ophthalmology. 3rd ed. Philadelphia: Saunders/Elsevier; 2008. p. 3749.
14. Miller FW. Myositis-specific autoantibodies: touchstones for understanding the inflammatory myopathies. JAMA. 1993;270:1846–9.
15. Lakhanpal S, Bunch TW, Ilstrup DM, et al. Polymyositis-dermatomyositis and malignant lesions: does an associa-tion exist? Mayo Clin Proc. 1986;61:645–53.
16. Vleugels RA, Callen JP. Dermatomyositis. In: Lebwohl MG, editor. Treatment of skin disease: comprehensive therapeutic strategies. 5th ed. Frisco: Elsevier; 2018. p. 198–202.
17. Shaikh MF, Jordan N, D'Cruz DP. Systemic lupus erythematous. Clin Med (Lond). 2017 Feb;17(1):78–83. https://doi.org/10.7861/clinmedicine.17-1-78.
18. Somers EC, Marder W, Cagnoli P, et al. Population-based incidence and prevalence of systemic lupus erythemato-sus: the Michigan lupus epidemiology and surveillance program: incidence and prevalence of SLE in southeastern Michigan. Arthritis Rheumatol. 2014;66:369–78.
19. Foster CS, Sobrin L. Systemic lupus erythematous. In: Albert M, et al., editors. Albert & Jakobiec's Principles and Practice of Ophthalmology. 3rd ed. Philadelphia: Saunders/Elsevier; 2008. p. 4429–36.
20. Pathak S, Mohan C. Cellular and molecular pathogenesis of systemic lupus erythematosus: lessons from animal models. Arthritis Res Ther. 2011;13:241.
21. Purdy EP, Bolling JP, Di Lorenzo AL, et al. Rheumatic disorders. In: Update on general medicine. Section 1, Basic and clinical science course. Philadelphia: American Academy of Ophthalmology. 2010–2011 ed. p. 167–70.
22. Ruiz-Irastorza G, Garcia M, Espinosa G, et al. First month prednisone dose predicts prednisone burden during the following 11 months: an observational study from the RELES cohort. Lupus Sci Med. 2016;3:e000153.
23. Houssiau FA, Vasconcelos C, D'Cruz D, et al. Immunosuppressive therapy in lupus nephritis: the Euro-Lupus Nephritis Trial, a randomized trial of low-dose versus high-dose intravenous cyclophosphamide. Arthritis Rheum. 2002;46(8):2121–31.
24. Yasuda S. Emerging targets for the treatment of lupus erythematosus: there is no royal road to treating lupus. Mod Rheumatol. 2019;29(1):60–9. https://doi.org/10.1080/14397595.2018.1493909.
25. Barnes J, Mayes MD. Epidemiology of systemic sclerosis: incidence, prevalence, survival, risk factors, malignancy, and environmental triggers. Curr Opin Rheumatol. 2012;24(2):165–70. https://doi.org/10.1097/BOR.0b013e32834ff2e8.
26. Dana R, Chong EV, Forster CS. Scleroderma. In: Albert M, et al., editors. Albert & Jakobiec's principles and practice of ophthalmology. 3rd ed. Philadelphia: Saunders/Elsevier; 2008. p. 4461–8.
27. Purdy EP, Bolling JP, Di Lorenzo AL, et al. Rheumatic disorders. In: Update on general medicine. Section 1, Basic and clinical science course. San Francisco: American Academy of Ophthalmology. 2010–2011 ed. p. 173–74.
28. Subcommittee for Scleroderma Criteria of the American Rheumatism Association Diagnostic and Therapeutic Criteria Committee: Preliminary Criteria for the classification of systemic sclerosis (scleroderma). Arthritis Rheum. 1980;23:581–90.
29. Ferreli C, Gasparini G, Parodi A, Cozzani E, Rongioletti F, Atzori L. Cutaneous manifestations of scleroderma and scleroderma-like disorders: a comprehensive review. Clin Rev Allerg Immunol. 2017;53:306–36. https://doi.org/10.1007/s12016-017-8625-4.
30. Mouthon L, Bussone G, Berezné A, Noël LH, Guillevin L. Scleroderma renal crisis. J Rheumatol. 2014;41:1040–8.
31. Pope JE, Bellamy N, Seibold JR, et al. A randomized, con- trolled trial of methotrexate versus placebo in early diffuse sclero-derma. Arthritis Rheum. 2001;44:1351–8.
32. Rubio-Rivas M, Royo C, Simeón CP, Corbella X, Fonollosa V. Mortality and survival in systemic sclerosis: sys-tematic review and meta-analysis. Semin Arthritis Rheum. 2014;44:208–19.
33. Maciel G, Crowson CS, Matteson EL, Cornec D. Prevalence of primary Sjogren's syndrome in a population- based cohort in the United States. Arthritis Care Res (Hoboken). 2016; https://doi.org/10.1002/acr.23173.
34. Efe C, Wahlin S, Ozaslan E, Berlot AH, Purnak T, Muratori L, Quarneti C, Yuksel O, Thiefin G, Muratori P. Autoimmune hepatitis/primary biliary cirrhosis overlap syndrome and associated extrahepatic autoimmune dis-eases. Eur J Gastroenterol Hepatol. 2012;24(5):531–4. https://doi.org/10.1097/MEG.0b013e328350f95b.

35. Haacke EA, Bootsma H, Spijkervet FKL, Visser A, Vissink A, Kluin PM, Kroese FGM. FcRL4+ B-cells in salivary glands of primary Sjogren's syndrome patients. J Autoimmun. 2017;81:90–8. https://doi.org/10.1016/j.jaut.2017.03.012.
36. Purdy EP, Bolling JP, Di Lorenzo AL, et al. Rheumatic disorders. In: External disease and cornea, basic and clinical science course. San Francisco: American Academy of Ophthalmology. 2010–2011 ed. p. 63–5.
37. Bernacchi E, Bianchi B, Amato L, Giorgini S, Fabbri P, Tavoni A, Bombardieri S. Xerosis in primary Sjogren syndrome: immunohistochemical and functional investigations. J Dermatol Sci. 2005;39(1):53–5. https://doi.org/10.1016/j.jdermsci.2005.01.017.
38. Ramos-Casals M, Brito-Zeron P, Seror R, Bootsma H, Bowman SJ, Dorner T, Gottenberg JE, Mariette X, Theander E, Bombardieri S, De Vita S, Mandl T, Ng WF, Kruize A, Tzioufas A, Vitali C, Force ESST. Characterization of systemic disease in primary Sjogren's syndrome: EULAR-SS task force recommendations for articular, cutaneous, pulmonary and renal involvements. Rheumatology (Oxford). 2015;54(12):2230–8. https://doi.org/10.1093/rheumatology/kev200.
39. Lawley TJ, Moutsopoulos HM, Katz SI, Theofilopoulos AN, Chused TM, Frank MM. Demonstration of circulating immune complexes in Sjogren's syndrome. J Immunol. 1979;123(3):1382–7.
40. Katayama I, Koyano T, Nishioka K. Prevalence of eyelid dermatitis in primary Sjogren's syndrome. Int J Dermatol. 1994;33(6):421–4.
41. Rischmueller M, Tieu J, Lester S. Primary Sjogren's syndrome. Best Pract Res Clin Rheumatol. 2016;30(1):189–220. https://doi.org/10.1016/j.berh.2016.04.003.
42. Shen L, Suresh L. Autoantibodies, detection methods and panels for diagnosis of Sjogren's syndrome. Clin Immunol. 2017; https://doi.org/10.1016/j.clim.2017.03.017.
43. Judson MA. The clinical features of sarcoidosis: a comprehensive review. Clinic Rev Allergy Immunol. 2015;49:63–78. https://doi.org/10.1007/s12016-014-8450.
44. Arkema EV, Cozier YC. Epidemiology of sarcoidosis: current findings and future directions. Ther Adv Chronic Dis. 2018;9(11):227–40. https://doi.org/10.1177/2040622318790197.
45. Prasse A, Katic C, Germann M, et al. Phenotyping sarcoidosis from a pulmonary perspective. Am J Respir Crit Care Med. 2008;177:330–6.
46. Lynch JP 3rd, Kazerooni EA, Gay SE. Pulmonary sarcoidosis. Clin Chest Med. 1997;18:755–85.
47. Scadding JG. Prognosis of intrathoracic sarcoidosis in England. A review of 136 cases after five years' observation. Br Med J. 1961;2:1165–72.
48. Purdy EP, Bolling JP, Di Lorenzo AL, et al. Noninfectious (autoimmune) uveitis. In: Intraocular inflammation and uveitis, basic and clinical science course. San Francisco: American Academy of Ophthalmology. 2010–2011 ed. p. 199–204.
49. Jabs DA, Johns CJ. Ocular involvement in chronic sarcoidosis. Am J Ophthalmol. 1986;102:297–301.
50. Aubart FC, Ouayoun M, Brauner M, et al. Sinonasal involvement in sarcoidosis: a case–control study of 20 patients. Medicine (Baltimore). 2006;85:365–71.
51. Neville E, Walker AN, James DG. Prognostic factors predicting the outcome of sarcoidosis: an analysis of 818 patients. Q J Med. 1983;52:525–33.
52. Eklund A, Rizzato G. Skin manifestations in sarcoidosis. Eur Resp J Monog. 2005;10:150–63.
53. Kim EC, Forster CS. Systyemic manifestations of sarcoidosis. In: Albert M, et al., editors. Albert & Jakobiec's principles and practice of ophthalmology. 3rd ed. Philadelphia: Saunders/Elsevier; 2008. p. 4483–94.
54. Rajput R, Mathewson P, Mudhar HS, et al. Periocular cutaneous sarcoid: case series and review of the literature. Eye. 2019;33:1590–5. https://doi.org/10.1038/s41422-019-0448-5.
55. Demirci H, Christianson MD. Orbital and adnexal involvement in sarcoidosis: analysis of clinical features and systemic disease in 30 cases. Am J Ophthalmol. 2011;151:1074–80.
56. Valeyre D, Prasse A, Nunes H, Uzunhan Y, Brillet PY, Müller-Quernheim J. Sarcoidosis. Lancet. 2014;383(9923):1155–67. https://doi.org/10.1016/S0140-6736(13)60680-7. Epub 2013 Oct 1
57. Tan J, Berg M. Rosacea: current state of epidemiology. J Am Acad Dermatol. 2013;69(6 Suppl 1):S27–35.
58. Spoendlin J, Voegel JJ, Jick SS, Meier CR. A study on the epidemiology of rosacea in the U.K. Br J Dermatol. 2012;167:598–605. https://doi.org/10.1111/j.1365-2133.2012.11037.x. PMID:22564022
59. Two AM, Wu W, Gallo RL, Hata TR. Rosacea: part I. Introduction, categorization, histology, pathogenesis, and risk factors. J Am Acad Dermatol. 2015;72:749–58. https://doi.org/10.1016/j.jaad.2014.08.028, PMID:25890455
60. Purdy EP, Bolling JP, Di Lorenzo AL, et al. Ocular surface disease: diagnostic approach. In: External disease and cornea, basic and clinical science course. San Francisco: American Academy of Ophthalmology. 2010–2011 ed. p. 69–71.
61. Koller B, Muller-Wiefel AS, Rupec R, Korting HC, Ruzicka T. Chitin modulates innate immune responses of keratinocytes. PLoS One. 2011;6:e16594.

62. Jang YH, Sim JH, Kang HY, Kim YC, Lee ES. Immuno- histochemical expression of matrix metalloproteinases in the granulomatous rosacea compared with the non-granulomatous rosacea. J Eur Acad Dermatol Venereol. 2011;25:544–8.

63. Szlachcic A. The link between Helicobacter pylori infection and rosacea. J Eur Acad Dermatol Venereol. 2002;16:328–33.

64. Wanke I, Steffen H, Christ C, et al. Skin commensals amplify the innate immune response to pathogens by activation of distinct signaling pathways. J Invest Dermatol. 2011;131:382–90.

65. Pelle MT, Crawford GH, James WD. Rosacea: II. Therapy. J Am Acad Dermatol. 2004;51:499–512.

66. Two AM, Wu W, Gallo RL, Hata TR. Rosacea: part II. Topical and systemic therapies in the treatment of rosacea. J Am Acad Dermatol. 2015;72:761–70; quiz 71–2. https://doi.org/10.1016/j.jaad.2014.08.027. PMID:25890456.

67. Schwartz JR, Cardin CW, Dawson TL. Seborrheic dermatitis and dandruff. In: Baran R, Maibach HI, editors. Textbook of cosmetic dermatology. London: Martin Dunitz, Ltd; 2010. p. 230–41.

68. Sampaio AL, Mameri AC, Vargas TJ, Ramos-e-Silva M, Nunes AP, et al. Seborrheic dermatitis. An Bras Dermatol. 2011;86:1061–71.

69. Borda LJ, Wikramanayake TC. Seborrheic Dermatitis and Dandruff: A Comprehensive Review. J Clin Investig Dermatol. 2015;3(2) https://doi.org/10.13188/2373-1044.1000019.

70. Faergemann J. Treatment of seborrhoeic dermatitis of the scalp with ketoconazole shampoo. A double-blind study. Acta Derm Venereol. 1990;70(2):171–2.

71. Okada K, Endo Y, Fujisawa A, Tanioka M, Kabashima K, et al. Refractory seborrheic dermatitis of the head in a patient with malignant lymphoma. Case Rep Dermatol. 2014;6:279–82.

72. Dunic I, Vesic S, Jevtovic DJ. Oral candidiasis and seborrheic dermatitis in HIV-infected patients on highly active antiretroviral therapy. HIV Med. 2004;5:50–4.

73. Schwartz JR, Messenger AG, Tosti A, et al. A comprehensive pathophysiology of dandruff and seborrheic dermatitis – towards a more precise definition of scalp health. Acta Derm Venereol. 2013;93(2):131–7.

74. Del Rosso JQ. Adult seborrheic dermatitis: a status report on practical topical management. J Clin Aesthet Dermatol. 2011;4:32–8.

75. Purdy EP, Bolling JP, Di Lorenzo AL, et al. Ocular surface disease: diagnostic approach. In: External disease and cornea, basic and clinical science course. American Academy of Ophthalmology. 2010–2011 ed. p. 71–3.

76. Waldroup W, Scheinfeld N. Medicated shampoos for the treatment of seborrheic dermatitis. J Drugs Dermatol. 2008;7(7):699–703.

77. Piérard-Franchimont C, Piérard GE, Arrese JE, De Doncker P. Effect of ketoconazole 1% and 2% shampoos on severe dandruff and sebor- rhoeic dermatitis: clinical, squamometric and mycological assessments. Dermatology. 2001;202(2):171–6.

78. Ang-Tiu CU, Meghrajani CF, Maano CC. Pimecrolimus 1% cream for the treatment of seborrheic dermatitis: a systematic review of randomized controlled trials. Expert Rev Clin Pharmacol. 2012;5(1):91–7.

79. Drucker AM, Wang AR, Li WQ, Sevetson E, Block JK, Qureshi AA. The burden of atopic dermatitis: summary of a report for the National Eczema Association. J Invest Dermatol. 2017;137(1):26–30. https://doi.org/10.1016/j.jid.2016.07.012.

80. Nutten S. Atopic dermatitis: global epidemiology and risk factors. Ann Nutr Metab. 2015;66(suppl 1):8–16. https://doi.org/10.1159/000370220.

81. Eichenfield LF, Tom WL, Chamlin SL, et al. Guidelines of care for the management of atopic dermatitis: section 1. Diagnosis and assessment of atopic dermatitis. J Am Acad Dermatol. 2014;70(2):338–51. https://doi.org/10.1016/j.jaad.2013.10.010.

82. Ozkaya E. Adult-onset atopic dermatitis. J Am Acad Dermatol. 2005;52(4):579–82.

83. Kim JP, Chao LX, Simpson EL, Silverberg JI. Persistence of atopic dermatitis (AD): a systematic review and meta-analysis. J Am Acad Dermatol. 2016;75(4):681–687.e11. https://doi.org/10.1016/j.jaad.2016.05.028.

84. Silverberg NB, Silverberg JI. Inside out or outside in: does atopic dermatitis disrupt barrier function or does disruption of barrier function trigger atopic dermatitis? Cutis. 2015;96(6):359–61.

85. Avena-Woods C. Overview of atopic dermatitis. Am J Manag Care. 2017;23(8 Suppl):S115–23.

86. Hanifin JM, Rajka G. Diagnostic features of atopic dermatitis. Acta Derm Venereol (Stockh). 1980;92(suppl):44–7.

87. Eichenfield LF, Hanifin JM, Luger TA, Stevens SR, Pride HB. Consensus conference on pediatric atopic dermatitis. J Am Acad Dermatol. 2003;49(6):1088–95. https://doi.org/10.1067/S0190.

88. Purdy EP, Bolling JP, Di Lorenzo AL, et al. Clinical approach to immune-related disorders of the external eye. In: External disease and cornea, basic and clinical science course. San Francisco: American Academy of Ophthalmology. 2010–2011 ed. p. 185.

89. Chisholm SAM, Couch SM, Custer PL. Etiology and management of allergic conjunctivitis. Ophthal Plast Reconstr Surg. 2017;33(4):248–50. https://doi.org/10.1097/IOP0000000000000723.

90. Eichenfield LF, Tom WT, Berger TG, et al. Guidelines of care for the management of atopic dermatitis. Part 2. J Am Acad Dermatol. 2014;71:116–32.

91. Sidbury R, Kodama S. Atopic dermatitis guidelines: diagnosis, systemic therapy, and adjunctive care. Clin Dermatol. 2018;36:648–52. https://doi.org/10.1016/j.clindermatol.2018.05.008.

92. Silverberg NB. A practical overview of pediatric atopic dermatitis, part 1: epidemiology and pathogenesis. Cutis. 2016;97(4):267–71.

93. Totri CP, Eichenfield LF, Logan K, et al. Prescribing practices for sys- temic agents in the treatment of severe pediatric atopic dermatitis in the US and Canada: the PeDRA TREAT survey. J Am Acad Dermatol. 2017;76:281–5.

94. Seegräber M, Srour J, Walter A, Knop M, Wollenberg A. Dupilumab for treatment of atopic dermatitis. Expert Rev Clin Pharmacol. 2018;11(5):467–74. https://doi.org/10.1080/17512433.2018.1449642.

95. Vahlquist A, Fischer J, Torma H. Inherited nonsyndromic ichthyoses: an update on pathophysiology, diagnosis and treatment. Am J Clin Dermatol. 2018;19:51–66. https://doi.org/10.1007/s40257-017-0313-x.

96. Schmuth M, Gruber R, Elias PM, Williams ML. Ichthyosis update: towards a function-driven model of pathogenesis of the disorders of cornification and the role of corneocyte proteins in these disorders. Adv Dermatol. 2007;23:231–56.

97. Sadowski AE. Dermatologic disorders and the cornea. In: Krachmer JH, Mannis MJ, Holland EJ, editors. Cornea. 3rd ed: Mosby/Elsevier; 2011. p. 755–7.

98. Shwayder T, Ott F. All about ichthyosis. Pediatr Clin N Am. 1991;38:835–57.

99. Malhotra R, Hernández-Martın A, Oji V. Br J Ophthalmol. 2018;102:586–92. https://doi.org/10.1136/bjophthalmol-2017-310615.

100. Cruz AA, Menezes FA, Chaves R, et al. Eyelid abnormalities in lamellar ichthyoses. Ophthalmology. 2000;107:1895–8.

101. Takeichi T, Akiyama M. Inherited ichthyosis: non-syndromic forms. J Dermatol. 2016;43(3):242–51.

102. Zhou Y, Liu J, Cui Y, et al. Moisture chamber versus lubrication for corneal protection in critically ill patients: a meta-analysis. Cornea. 2014;33:1179–85.

103. Leung PC, Ma GF. Ectropion of all four eyelids associated with severe ichthyosis congenita: a case report. Br J Plast Surg. 1981;34:302–4.

104. Deffenbacher B. Successful experimental treatment of congenital ichthyosis in an infant. BMJ Case Rep. March 6; 2013:bcr2013008688.

105. Taban M, Mancini R, Nakra T, et al. Nonsurgical management of congenital eyelid malpositions using hyaluronic acid gel. Ophthal Plast Reconstr Surg. 2009;25:259–63.

106. Shikari H, Antin JH, Dana R. Ocular graft-versus-host disease: a review. Surv Ophthalmol. 2013;58:233–51.

107. Uchino M, Ogawa Y, Uchino Y, et al. Comparison of stem cell sources in the severity of dry eye after allogeneic haematopoietic stem cell transplantation. Br J Ophthalmol. 2012;96:34–7.

108. Eapen M, Logan BR, Confer DL, et al. Peripheral blood grafts from unrelated donors are associated with increased acute and chronic graft-versus-host disease without improved survival. Biol Blood Marrow Transplant. 2007;13:1461–8.

109. Ferrara JL, Levine JE, Reddy P, et al. Graft-versus-host disease. Lancet. 2009;373:1550–61.

110. Kim SK. Ocular graft-versus-host disease. In: Krachmer JH, Mannis MJ, Holland EJ, editors. Cornea. 3rd ed. Maryland Heights: Mosby/Elsevier; 2011. p. 789–96.

111. Vogelsang GB, Lee L, Bensen-Kennedy DM. Pathogenesis and treatment of graft-versus-host disease after bone marrow transplant. Annu Rev Med. 2003;54:29–52.

112. Hirst LW, Jabs DA, Tutschka PJ, et al. The eye in bone marrow transplantation. I Clinical study. Arch Ophthalmol. 1983;101:580–4.

113. Ramachandran V, Kolli SS, Strowd LC. Review of graft-versus-host disease. Dermatol Clin. 2019;37:569–82. https://doi.org/10.1016/j.det.2019.05.014.

114. Anderson NG, Regillo C. Ocular manifestations of graft versus host disease. Curr Opin Ophthalmol. 2004;15:503–7.

115. Ogawa Y, Yamazaki K, Kuwana M, et al. A significant role of stromal fibroblasts in rapidly progressive dry eye in patients with chronic GVHD. Invest Ophthalmol Vis Sci. 2001;42:111–9.

116. Kim SK, Couriel D, Ghosh S, et al. Ocular graft vs. host disease experience from MD Anderson Cancer Center: newly described clinical spectrum and new approach to the management of stage III and IV ocular GVHD. Biol Blood Marrow Transplant. 2006;12:49–50.

117. Campbell AA, Jakobiec FA, Rashid A, et al. Bilateral sequential dacryocystitis &&in a patient with graft-versus-host disease. Ophthal Plast Reconstr Surg. 2016;32:e89–92.

118. Johnson DA, Jabs DA. The ocular manifestations of graft-versus-Uhost disease. N Engl J Med. 1992;326:1055–8.

119. Martin PJ, Schoch G, Fisher L, et al. A retrospective analysis of therapy for acute graft-versus-host disease: secondary treatment. Blood. 1991;77:1821–8.

120. Greinix HT, Knobler RM, Worel N, et al. The effect of intensified extracorporeal photochemotherapy on long-term survival in patients with severe acute graft-versus-host disease. Haematologica. 2006;91:405–8.

121. Russo PA, Bouchard CS, Galasso JM. Extended-wear silicone hydrogel soft contact lenses in the management of moderate to severe dry eye signs and symptoms secondary to graft-versus-host disease. Eye Contact Lens. 2007;33:144.

122. Shay E, Kheirkhah A, Liang L, Sheha H, Gregory DG, Tseng SCG. Amniotic membrane transplantation as a new therapy for the acute ocular manifestations of Stevens-Johnson syndrome and toxic epidermal necrolysis. Surv Ophthalmol. 2009;54:686–96.

123. Rocha EM, Pelegrino FS, de Paiva CS, et al. GVHD dry eyes treated with autologous serum tears. Bone Marrow Transpl. 2000;25:1101–3.

124. Smith VA, Cook SD. Doxycycline-a role in ocular surface repair. Br J Ophthalmol. 2004;88:619–25.

125. Takahide K, Parker PM, Wu M, et al. Use of fluid-ventilated, gas-permeable scleral lens for management of severe keratoconjunctivitis sicca secondary to chronic graft- versus-host disease. Biol Blood Marrow Transplant. 2007;13:1016–21.

126. Bonidas JM, Rothman AL, Spstein EH. Epidermolysis bullosa simplex: evidence in two families for keratin gene abnormalities. Science. 1991;254:1202–5.

127. Coulombe PA, Hutton ME, Letai A, et al. Point mutations in human keratin 14 genes of epidermolysis bullosa simplex patients: genetic and functional analyzes. Cell. 1991;66:1301–11.

128. Marinkovich MP. The molecular genetics of basement membrane diseases. Arch Dermatol. 1993;129:1557–65.

129. Uitto J, Pulkkinen L, Christiano AM. Molecular basis of the dystrophic and junctional form of epidermolysis bullosa: mutations in the type VII collagen and kalinin (laminin-5) genes. J Invest Dermatol. 1994;103(5 Suppl):S39–46.

130. Pai S, Marinkovich MP. Epidermolysis Bullosa: new and emerging trends. Am J Clin Dermatol. 2002;3(6):371–80. 1175–0561

131. Sadowsky AE. Dermatologic disorders and the cornea. In: Krachmer JH, Mannis MJ, Holland EJ, editors. Cornea. 3rd ed. Maryland Heights: Mosby/Elsevier; 2011. p. 749–61.

132. Mellado F, Fuentes I, Palisson F, Vergara JI, Kantor A. Ophthalmic approach in epidermolysis bullosa: a cross-sectional study with phenotype-genotype correlations. Cornea. 2018;37:442–7.

133. Ruocco V, Ruocco E, Lo Schiavo A, et al. Pemphigus: etiology, pathogenesis, and inducing or triggering factors: facts and controversies. Clin Dermatol. 2013;31:374–81.

134. Chirinos-Saldana P, Nava A, Ramirez-Miranda A, Jimenez-Martinez MC, Graue-Hernandez EO. Pemphigus: an ophthalmological review. Eye Contact Lens. 2016;42:91–8. https://doi.org/10.1097/ICL.0000000000000155.

135. Joly P, Litrowski N. Pemphigus group (vulgaris, vegetans, foliaceus, herpetiformis, brasiliensis). Clin Dermatol. 2011;29:432–6.

136. Becker BA, Gaspari AA. Pemphigus vulgaris and vegetans. Dermatol Clin. 1993;11:429–52.

137. Sadowsky AE. Dermatologic disorders and the cornea. In: Krachmer JH, Mannis MJ, Holland EJ, editors. Cornea. 3rd ed. Maryland Heights: Mosby/Elsevier; 2011. p. 752.

138. Kaplan I, Hodak E, Ackerman L, et al. Neoplasms associated 580 with paraneoplastic pemphigus: a review with emphasis on non-hematologic malignancy and oral mucosal manifestations. Oral Oncol. 2004;40:553–62.

139. Meyers SJ, Varley GA, Meisler DM, et al. Conjunctival involvement in paraneoplastic pemphigus. Am J Ophthalmol. 1992;114:621–4.

140. Pisani M, Ruocco V. Drug-induced pemphigus. Clin Dermatol. 1986;4:118–32.

141. Venugopal SS, Murrell DF. Diagnosis and clinical features of pemphigus vulgaris. Immunol Allergy Clin N Am. 2012;32:233–43. v–vi

142. Baykal HE, Pleyer U, Sonnichsen K, et al. Severe eye involvement in pemphigus vulgaris [in German]. Ophthalmologe. 1995;92:854–7.

143. Daoud YJ, Foster CS, Ahmed R. Eyelid skin involvement in pemphigus foliaceus. Ocul Immunol Inflamm. 2005;13:389–94.

144. Kasperkiewicz M, Schmidt E, Zillikens D. Current therapy of the pemphigus group. Clin Dermatol. 2012;30:84–94.

145. Wang HH, Liu CW, Li YC, Huang YC. Efficacy of rituximab for pemphigus: a systematic review and meta-analysis of different regimens. Acta Derm Venereol. 2015;95(8):928–32. https://doi.org/10.2340/00015555-2116.

146. Tam PM, Cheng LL, Young AL, Lam PT. Paraneoplastic pemphigus: an uncommon cause of chronic cicatrising conjunctivitis. BMJ Case Rep. 2009. doi:10.1136/bcr.12.2008.1306

147. Chiou AG, Florakis GJ, Kazim M. Management of conjunctival cicatrizing diseases and severe ocular surface dysfunction. Surv Ophthalmol. 1998;43:19–46.

148. Laforest C, Huilgol SC, Casson R, et al. Autoimmune bullous diseases: ocular manifestations and management. Drugs. 2005;65:1767–79.

149. Ruocco E, Sangiuliano S, Gravina AG, Miranda A, Nicoletti G. Pyoderma gangrenosum: an updated review. J Eur Acad Dermatol Venereol. 2009;23:1008–17.

150. Adachi Y, Kindzelskii AL, Cookingham G, et al. Aberrant neutrophil trafficking and metabolic oscillations in severe pyoderma gangrenosum. J Invest Dermatol. 1998;111:259–68.

151. Callen JP. Pyoderma gangrenosum. Lancet. 1998;351:581–5.

152. Binus AM, Qureshi AA, Li VW, Winterfield LS. Pyoderma gangrenosum: a retrospective review of patient characteristics, comorbidities and therapy in 103 patients. Br J Dermatol. 2011;165:1244–50.

153. Powell FC, Schroeter AL, Su WP, Perry HO. Pyoderma gangrenosum: a review of 86 patients. Q J Med. 1985;55:173–86.
154. Gupta AS, Ortega-Loayza AG. Ocular pyoderma Gangrenosum: a systematic review. J Am Acad Dermatol. 2017;76:512–7.
155. Wollina U. Clinical management of pyoderma gangrenosum. Am J Clin Dermatol. 2002;3:149–58.
156. Ye MJ, Ye JM. Pyoderma gangrenosum: a review of clinical features and outcomes of 23 cases requiring inpatient management. Dermatol Res Pract. 2014;2014:461467.
157. Moynahan EJ. Acrodermatitis enteropathica: a lethal inherited human zinc deficiency disorder. Lancet. 1974;2:399–400.
158. Lucky AW. Cutaneous manifestations of endocrine, metabolic, and nutritional disorders. In: Schachner LA, Hansen RC, editors. Pediatric dermatology. New York: Churchill Livingstone; 1995. p. 1077–80.
159. Fraker JP, Jardieu P, Cook J. Zinc deficiency and immune function. Arch Dermatol. 1987;123:1698–700.
160. Perafan-Riveros C, Franca LFS, Alves ACF, Sanches JA Jr. Acrodermatitis Enteropathica: case report and review of the literature. Pediatr Dermatol. 2002;19:426–31.
161. Moynahan EJ, Barnes KM. Zinctherapyinasyntheticdiet for lactose intolerance. Lancet. 1973;1:676–7.
162. Lee MG, Hong KT, Kim JJ. Transient symptomatic zinc deficiency in a full term breast-fed infant. J Am Acad Dermatol. 1990;23:375–9.
163. Post CF, Juhlin E. Demodex folliculorum blepharitis. Arch Dermatol. 1963;88:298–302.
164. English FP, Nutting WB. Demodicosis of ophthalmic concern. Am J Ophthalmol. 1981;91:362–72.
165. Liang L, Ding X, Tseng SC. High prevalence of Demodex brevis infestation in chalazia. Am J Ophthalmol. 2014;157:342–8.
166. Kheirkhah A, Casas V, Li W, et al. Corneal manifestations of ocular Demodex infestation. Am J Ophthalmol. 2007;143:743–9.
167. Li J, O'Reilly N, Sheha H, et al. Correlation between ocular Demodex infestation and serum immunoreactivity to Bacillus proteins in patients with facial rosacea. Ophthalmology. 2010;117:870–7.
168. Gao YY, Di Pascuale MA, Elizondo A, Tseng SC. Clinical treatment of ocular demodecosis by lid scrub with tea tree oil. Cornea. 2007;26:136–43.
169. Tighe S, Gao YY, Tseng SC. Terpinen-4-ol is the most active ingredient of tea tree oil to kill mites. Transl Vis Sci Technol. 2013;2:2.
170. Cheng AMS, Sheha H, Tseng SCG. Recent advances on ocular Demodex infestation. Curr Opin Ophthalmol. 2015;26:296–300. https://doi.org/10.1097/ICU.0000000000000168.
171. Park DJJ, Woog JJ, Glover AT. Eyelid infections. In: Albert, Miller et al. editors. Albert & Jakobiec's principles and practice of ophthalmology. 3rd Ed. Philadelphia: Saunders/Elsevier; 2008. pg 3229.
172. Purdy EP, Bolling JP, Di Lorenzo AL, et al. Infectious diseases/external eye: basic concepts and viral infections. In: External disease and cornea, basic and clinical science course. San Francisco: American Academy of Ophthalmology. 2010–2011 ed. p. 105–19.
173. Moyes AL, Verachtert AJ. Eyelid infections. In: Krachmer JH, Mannis MJ, Holland EJ editors. Cornea. 3rd Ed. Maryland Heights: Mosby/Elsevier, 2011. Pg 415.
174. Park DJJ, Woog JJ, Glover AT. Eyelid infections. In: Albert, Miller et al. editors. Albert & Jakobiec's principles and practice of ophthalmology. 3rd Ed. Philadelphia: Saunders/Elsevier, 2008.pg 3232–3233.
175. Moyes AL, Verachtert AJ. Eyelid infections. In: Krachmer JH, Mannis MJ, Holland EJ, editors. Cornea. 3rd ed. Maryland Heights: Mosby/Elsevier; 2011. p. 416–7.
176. Purdy EP, Bolling JP, Di Lorenzo AL, et al. Infectious diseases/external eye: basic concepts and viral infections. In: External disease and cornea, basic and clinical science course. 2010-112 ed. San Francisco: American Academy of Ophthalmology. p. 119–22.
177. Pavan-Langston D. Herpes zoster ophthalmicus. Neurology. 1995;45(Suppl 8):S58–60.

Diagnostic Tools

4

Roshni Vasaiwala, Clayton Kirk,
and Charles S. Bouchard

Introduction

Blepharitis is a common chronic ophthalmologic condition characterized by inflammation of the eyelid margins associated with symptoms of eye redness and irritation. It occurs in people of all ages, ethnicities, and in either sex. Classification schemes have included anatomic location, duration/chronicity, and etiology [1, 2]. The overlap of symptoms and signs and the association with dermatologic conditions including rosacea, seborrheic dermatitis, and eczema can lead to misdiagnosis, underreporting of the condition and variable management protocols with variable outcomes. More severe and chronic eyelid disease can be a risk factor for corneal inflammatory disease and associated vision loss. Many cases of chronic blepharitis are also associated with evaporative dry eye disease (EDED) and meibomian gland dysfunction (MGD) [3, 4].

The complex multifactorial nature of chronic blepharitis includes inflammatory, infectious, and allergic mechanisms. This demands a structured and comprehensive multi-step approach to the diagnostic evaluation of blepharitis utilizing both subjective and objective measures. The sequence of testing is also important and will be outlined in this chapter. Consideration must also be given to normal changes in the eyelid and ocular surface physiology that occurs with age [5, 6].

Definitions and Classification

The International Workshop on MGD in 2011 established the following definition of MGD: "a chronic, diffuse abnormality of the meibomian glands (MGs), commonly characterized by terminal duct obstruction and/or qualitative and quantitative changes in the glandular secretion, which may result in alteration of the tear film, symptoms of eye irritation, clinically apparent inflammation, and ocular surface disease" [2, 7].

Dry eye disease (DED) has also been defined as "a multifactorial disease of the ocular surface characterized by a loss of homeostasis of the tear film and accompanied by ocular symptoms in which

R. Vasaiwala · C. Kirk · C. S. Bouchard (✉)
Loyola University Medical Center, Department of Ophthalmology, Maywood, IL, USA
e-mail: cboucha@lumc.edu

© Springer Nature Switzerland AG 2021
A. V. Farooq, J. J. Reidy (eds.), *Blepharitis*, Essentials in Ophthalmology,
https://doi.org/10.1007/978-3-030-65040-7_4

tear film instability, hyperosmolarity, ocular surface inflammation and damage, and neurosensory abnormalities play etiological roles" [3].

The most current classification system comes from the International Workshop on MGD: in the report of the Definition and Classification Subcommittee, the term "blepharitis" refers to inflammation of the eyelid as a whole, whereas marginal blepharitis refers to inflammation of the lid margin and includes anterior and posterior blepharitis [1].

Anterior blepharitis refers to inflammation anterior to the gray line and is associated with eyelash inflammation often associated with squamous debris and collarettes. It can be further categorized as staphylococcal or seborrheic types [8]. Staphylococci may alter meibomian gland secretion and cause blepharitis via various mechanisms [9–11]. The seborrheic type is characterized by dandruff-like skin changes and greasy scales around the base of the eyelids [8–12].

Posterior blepharitis refers to inflammation associated with the posterior lid margin and may include meibomian gland dysfunction (MGD), conjunctival inflammation, and other causes [7, 13–20]. MGD describes a chronic and diffuse inflammation of the meibomian glands commonly associated with terminal duct obstruction and/or abnormalities of the meibum secreted. The new classification system proposed by the International Workshop on MGD differentiates the different MGD subgroups on the basis of the level of secretion (see below). Obstructive MGD is the most common and constitutes the focus of the overview of the pathophysiology of MGD discussed below. This also introduces the role of MGD in the pathophysiology of evaporative dry eye (EDE) [1] (see below).

Pathophysiology

Blepharitis is a complex disorder involving interplay between the eyelids, meibomian glands, ocular surface, and lacrimal gland [13]. Altered lipid composition in gland secretions leads to instability of the tear film [18]. The abnormal secretions also have both a direct toxic effect on the ocular surface [21]. Additionally, because the microbiota of the tear film is dependent upon proper meibomian gland function, a proliferation of pathogenic microbes takes place [17, 18, 22, 23]. The altered tear film integrity and the proliferation of these organisms lead to a generalized inflammation of the ocular surface. Long-term inflammation leads to gland dysfunction, hyper-keratinization, and fibrosis. Hyper-keratinization, therefore, is an early finding in patients with posterior blepharitis, and diagnosing and grading this change is critical to staging the severity of the disease [24, 25]. These changes result in worsening meibomian gland function, perpetuating the cycle (Fig. 4.1).

Underlying inflammatory skin conditions such as rosacea and seborrheic dermatitis may cause posterior blepharitis, though these conditions commonly occur in their absence [13, 14, 26]. Chronic infection may also play a role in posterior blepharitis, although it is less well studied than in anterior blepharitis [27]. Other possible causes of blepharitis include contact (allergic) dermatitis, eczema, and psoriasis. Contact blepharitis is an acute inflammatory reaction of the skin of the eyelids, usually occurring as a reaction to an irritant [5]. *Demodex folliculorum* and *Demodex brevis* have been associated with posterior blepharitis [10, 28].

Epilation of the eyelashes for microscopic examination to detect *Demodex* mites is warranted when the clinical presentation (e.g., presence of cylindrical dandruff or "sleeves" on the eyelashes) is suggestive of this diagnosis or when there is severe or refractory blepharitis [11]. This is done by placing the eyelashes on a glass slide and then examining the organism under a cover slip after a drop of fluorescein has been added.

The etiology and pathophysiology of blepharitis differ based on the type of eyelid inflammation (posterior versus anterior). However, there is considerable overlap between these categories (Table 4.1). The remainder of this chapter will focus predominantly on MGD and the diagnosis and evaluation of this condition.

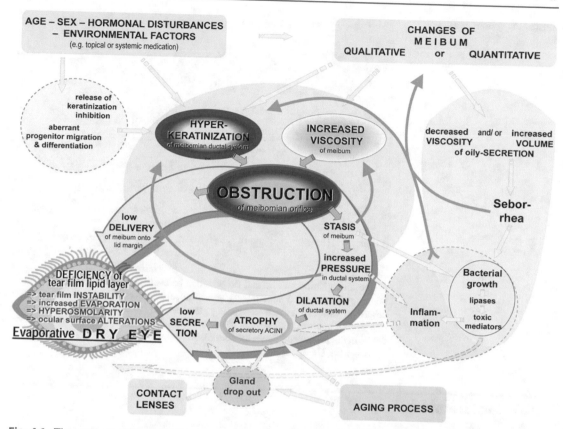

Fig. 4.1 The pathophysiologic cycle for meibomian gland dysfunction is a complex one. Multiple factors lead to obstruction and atrophy of the meibomian glands including inflammation, bacterial growth, aging, external factors including environment and contact lenses. (Nichols et al. [2])

Table 4.1 Techniques for imaging the meibomian glands

Technique	Lid region	Grading scheme
Meiboscopy	LL	0 = no dropout
		1 = ≤33%
		2 = 34–66%
		3 = ≥67%
		Percent of partial or total gland dropout
		Separate measurement over the nasal and temporal halves of the lower lid
Meibography (contact; retro-illumination)	LL	Total number of glands loss of eight central of the lower lid. Half gland loss was given a grade of 0.5
		1 = normal
		2 = gland visible w/decreased absorption
		3 = acini atrophic; duct visible
		4 = no structures visible
	LL	0 = no dropout
		1 = ≤50% dropout
		2 = ≥51% dropout
	LL	Dropout: (nasal half; lower eyelid)
		0 = no dropout
		1 = ≤25%

(continued)

Table 4.1 (continued)

Technique	Lid region	Grading scheme
		2 = ≤50%
		3 = ≤75%
		4 = ≤100%
	LL ≅ 15 glands	Gestalt method
		1 = no partial glands (PGs)
		2 = <25% PGs
		3 = 25–75% PGs
		4 = >75% PGs
Noncontact	LL and UL	0 = no loss,
		1 = gland loss <33% of total area
		2 = loss 33–66%
		3 = > 67% loss
		Scores of upper and lower lid summed Scale range: 0–6
Confocal microscopy	LL and/or UL	Acinar density: number of glands//mm² (based on 400 × 400 micrometer field) mean acinar diameter

Meibomian gland structure and dropout can be evaluated using meiboscopy, meibography (contact and noncontact), and confocal microscopy. Several authors have described various methods of grading gland atrophy and dropout based on these imaging techniques. References to the studies used to compose this table can be found in the referenced paper by Tomlinson et al. [29]
LL lower lid, *UL* upper lid

MGD: Background

Asymptomatic MGD is unknown to the patient but can be diagnosed by the clinician based on expression of the meibomian glands. With mechanical expression, there may be decreased or absent expression or the quality of material expressed may be abnormal.

As the disease progresses, it tends to become more symptomatic. In addition to typical dry eye symptoms, symptoms of MGD may include redness and swelling of the eyelid margins as well as irritation of the eyelid margins. At this stage, there are clinical signs that can be observed including meibomian gland dropout (meibography), changes in meibomian gland expression (thickness, volume, quality), and changes in eyelid morphology [29–32].

Meibomian gland dropout is diagnosed using the technique of meibography. This was first described by Mathers where the meibomian glands were evaluated on the mucosal side of the eyelid by transillumination of light applied to the skin side of the lid [33]. With age, the meibomian gland structure became less visible using this technique. The newer meibography techniques utilize infrared photography after eversion of the eyelids. Gland dropout can also be measured by confocal microscopy [34]. While meibomian gland dropout slowly increases with age even in normal patients, there can be more significant dropout in patients with MGD and worsening disease [31, 35, 36].

With MGD, expression of meibum, the material within the glands, can be altered in quantity and quality. Plugging of the meibomian glands can lead to decreased secretion of meibum on digital expression. Korb and Blackie [37] described standards for meibum secretion using a device that applies a standardized force on digital expression (Fig. 4.2). Quality of meibum expression can range from clear oil in normal patients to toothpaste-like material in patients with severe MGD. These can be quantified into various grading schemes (Table 4.1).

Changes in eyelid margin morphology are also noted in MGD. Plugging or pouting of the lids may be noted due to obstruction of the ducts and accumulation of lipid and keratinized cell debris at the

Fig. 4.2 Korb stimulator applies a standardize force to digitally express the meibomian glands and evaluate the quality of the meibomian gland oil. (Reference: Courtesy of Charles Bouchard, MD)

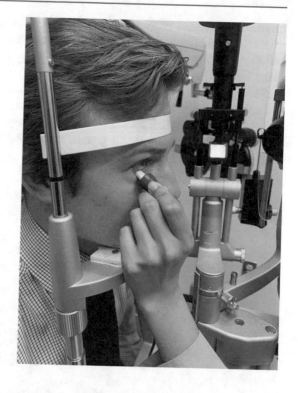

terminal ends. This has been identified as a pathognomonic clinical sign of MGD [25, 38]. The location of the meibomian gland openings in relation to the mucocutaneous junction and the location of the mucocutaneous junction within the lids can also be altered. In non-cicatricial MGD, the meibomian glands remain anterior to the mucocutaneous junction. With aging, the mucocutaneous junction moves anteriorly, thus making the gland orifices posterior to the junction. With cicatricial MGD, the orifices are displaced posteriorly across the mucocutaneous junction onto the conjunctiva. Cicatricial MGD can occur on its own, in conjunction with non-cicatricial MGD, or in association with other cicatrizing disorders such as trachoma and mucus membrane pemphigoid. Other eyelid structural features of MGD may include increased vascularity, telangiectasias, loss of gland opening architecture, cystic changes, concretions, and chalazia [37].

When clinically assessing MGD, grading scales have been developed to quantify gland dropout and quality of gland expression. As mentioned earlier, gland dropout can be measured by meiboscopy, meibography, and confocal microscopy. Meiboscopy utilizes lid transillumination with clinical observation, while meibography uses photo-documentation. Meibography is a more objective measure than meiboscopy [23, 25, 35].

Several grading scales have been developed and proposed using meiboscopy and meibography findings (Table 4.1). Pflugfelder et al. and others used a 0–3 scale and estimated partial or total gland loss in each of the nasal and temporal halves of the lid using meiboscopy [31, 39]. In this scale, 0 was no gland dropout, 1 was 1–33%, 2 was 34–66%, and 3 was greater than or equal to 67% dropout. Mathers et al. used meibography to measure the total number of glands lost within the central eight glands of the lower lid [40]. Fifty percent gland loss was given a grade of 0.5. Using meibography, Shimazaki et al. came up with a grading scale of 0–2 with 0 being no dropout, 1 < 50% dropout, and 2 being >50% dropout [41]. De Paiva et al. used a scale of 0 to 4 with 25% increased gland dropout at each level [42]. The study of Nichols et al. helped to validate the method of meibography and demonstrated repeatability and interobserver reliability of the technique [7]. Arita et al. used noncontact images to determine a score for each the lower and upper lids from 0 to 3 with 0 being no loss, 1 being <33% glans area loss, 2 being 33–67% loss, and 3 being >67% loss [24]. The score for each lid was summed, and the total score was known as the meiboscore. Image J can also be used to quantitate the gland loss [34].

Several grading scales have been developed to quantify the appearance of the expressed oil (Table 4.2 and Fig. 4.3). The scores in these systems are 0, clear; 1, cloudy; 2, cloudy with particles; 3, inspissated. Using these scales, there are two ways to calculate a score. One method uses the highest score measured for any of the glands. The second method uses a composite score, which is the sum

Table 4.2 Grading meibomian gland expression

Technique	Study details	Lid region	Grading scheme	Reference
Meibum characteristics				
Firm digital pressure	Volume of expressed meibum	Central eight glands of lower eyelid	0 = normal volume. Just covers orifice 1 = increased to 2 to 3 times normal 3 = increased more than 10 times	Mathers et al. [33]
Firm digital pressure	Viscosity of expressed meibum	Central eight glands of lower eyelid	1 = normal, clear, may have a few particles 2 = opaque with normal viscosity 3 = severe thickening (toothpaste)	Mathers et al. [33]
Firm digital pressure	Volume and viscosity of expressed meibum Clinic based; referred for dry eye or blepharitis $M = 513$ total; $N = 76$ normal women (used to define aqueous deficiency)	Central eight glands of lower eyelid	Obstructive: Viscosity ≥ 3 (1, clear; 2, slightly opaque; 3, thick, opaque; 4, toothpaste) Avg. lipid volume: ≤ 0.3 mm (diameter of expressed lipid in millimeters) Dropout: >0 (presumably examined central eight glands; includes 1/2 and whole glands) Seborrheic: Viscosity: no criteria Avg. lipid volume: >0.7 mm	Mathers et al. [33, 40]
Meibum quality and expressibility				
Firm digital pressure	Quality of meibum	Number of glands not stated UL or LL	0 = clear fluid 1 = cloudy fluid 2 = cloudy particulate fluid 3 = inspissated, like toothpaste	Bron et al. [83]
Firm digital pressure	Expressibility of meibum from five glands	UL or LL	0 = all glands expressible 1 = 3–4 glands expressible 2 = 1–2 glands expressible 3 = no glands expressible	Pflugfelder et al. [39]
Standardized application of pressure	Expression applied to a set of about eight glands	Nasal, central, and temporal lid	The MGYLS score is the number of meibomian glands out of 8, yielding liquid secretion	Korb and Blackie [37]
Meibum expressibility				
Variable digital pressure	Gentle or forceful expression	LL	Analysis of expressed secretion	Henriquez and Korb [85]
Variable digital pressure	Expressibility of meibum	LL	0 = clear meibum, easily expressed 1 = cloudy meibum, easily expressed 2 = cloudy meibum expressed with moderate pressure 3 = meibum not expressible, even with hard pressure	Shimazaki et al. [84]

Table 4.2 (continued)

Technique	Study details	Lid region	Grading scheme	Reference

Variable digital pressure using the Shimazaki schema	Measurement of lid morphology, expression, and meibography	See grading box	Lid margin:
			  Irregular
			  Vascular engorgement
			  Plugged orifices
			  Displacement of MCJ, score "1" for each present
				Arita et al. [86]

	Clinic based
	  $N = 53$ obstructive MGD subjects
	  $N = 60$ age-matched controls
			Expressed meibum (upper eyelid):
			  0 = clear, easily expressed
			  1 = cloudy, mild pressure
			  2 = cloudy, >moderate pressure
			  3 = meibum not expressed, with hard pressure	

			Meibography: upper and lower eyelids, meiboscore summed (0, no loss; 1, gland loss <33% of total area; 2, loss = 33–66%; 3, ≥67% loss)	

Several studies have looked at the quality and expressibility of meibomian gland oil using digital pressure and proposed various grading schemes. References to the studies used to compose this table can be found in the referenced paper by Tomlinson et al. [29]

of the scores for each gland expressed. The International Workshop Diagnosis Subcommittee recommends the latter method.

The expressibility of the glands has also been graded using a standard force applied to one or more glands [37]. Morphologic changes in the lids have also been graded in various ways, Arita et al. gave scores for the presence or absence of margin irregularity, lid margin vascular engorgement, orifice plugging, and anterior or retro-placement of the mucocutaneous junction, giving a score of 0–4 [24].

Clinical Evaluation and Diagnostic Testing

The following is a suggested standardized sequence of ocular surface clinical and diagnostic assessments, which should provide valuable diagnostic quantitative information to properly assess blepharitis and meibomian gland-related ocular surface disease.

Overview

1. Patient History
2. Review of Symptoms (ROS)
3. Symptom Questionnaire
4. Blink Rate (BR), Incomplete Blink Rate (IBR), Maximum Blink Interval (MBI)
5. External Examination
6. Tear Osmolarity
7. Meibography
8. Anterior Eye Assessment
9. Tear Film Assessment
10. Noninvasive Tear Breakup Time (NITBUT)
11. Tear Meniscus Height (TMH)

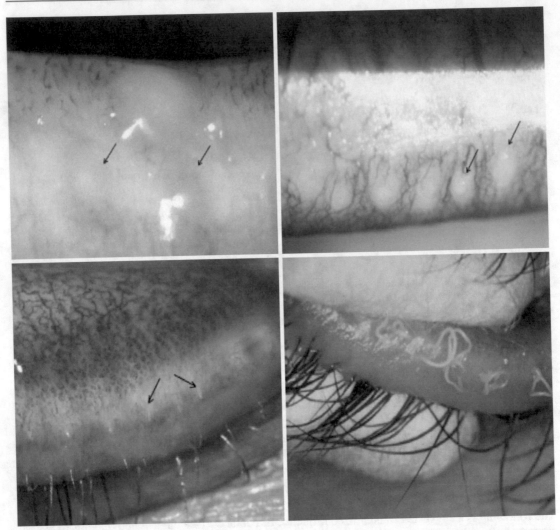

Fig. 4.3 Upper left: Cloudy expression of meibum. Upper right: Cicatricial meibomian gland dysfunction with lid margin telangiectasia and orifice occlusion. Lower left: Cicatricial meibomian gland dysfunction with posterior displacement of orifices. Lower right: Thickened "toothpaste-like" meibum. (Tomlinson et al. [29])

12. Tear Volume Assessment
13. Meibomian Gland Assessment
14. Corneal Integrity Assessment
15. Inflammatory Mediators

Patient History

Evaluation of a patient with possible blepharitis should always begin with careful and complete patient history and intake. Thorough patient history includes nature of ocular symptoms, timing, frequency, and triggers. It is imperative to understand what treatment modalities the patient has tried previously and whether or not these were successful [1, 13].

Review of Symptoms (ROS)

A careful review of systems and complete medication list is essential in determining the etiology of blepharitis and ocular surface disease. Prior medical history including history of diabetes mellitus, obstructive sleep apnea, autoimmune disease (rheumatoid arthritis, systemic lupus erythematosus, scleroderma, etc.) are important. Past surgical history, especially ocular surgical history, can play an important role in the diagnosis and management of blepharitis and eyelid disease. Refractive surgery, like blepharitis, has been shown to be a cause of dry eye disease. Medication use, especially those applied topically to the ocular surface, can contribute to poor eyelid hygiene and blepharitis [43, 44]. Social history, namely that of smoking history, may also be an important contributor to the blepharitis disease process [45].

Symptom Questionnaires (OSDI, DEQ-5, SPEED)

Questionnaires that measure the patient's perception of ocular surface discomfort and visual discomfort can be very helpful when evaluating patients with possible blepharitis. These can be filled out by the patient at the start of the clinic visit or in the waiting room prior to the visit. These symptom screening surveys can help confirm that a patient has dry eye disease and signal the technician and physician to perform the battery of diagnostic tests for this condition. There are several validated questionnaires that focus on the patient's self-reported symptoms [46, 47]. However, these questionnaires are not designed to distinguish between different types of ocular surface diseases.

Ocular Surface Disease Index (OSDI)

This standardized and frequently used survey includes 12 questions aimed to elicit symptoms related to ocular surface irritation, environmental triggers for the symptoms, and the effects on visual function in daily life [48]. The OSDI can quantify the frequency and impact of the symptoms on vision to assess disease severity. Total points vary from 0 to 100, with increasing numbers signifying greater symptom burden (normal <12; mild 12–21; moderate 22–33; severe >33) [5].

Dry Eye Questionnaire 5 (DEQ-5)

This survey includes only 5 items and has also been validated. DEQ-5 asks five questions regarding the frequency of watery eyes, discomfort, and dryness as well as late day intensity of discomfort and dryness. Scores >6 suggest dry eye and scores >12 may suggest more severe disease (Sjogren syndrome) [49].

Standard Patient Evaluation of Eye Dryness (SPEED)

The SPEED questionnaire is another validated dry eye survey that can be taken quickly, as its name suggests, SPEED evaluates the type, frequency, and severity of dry eye symptoms. The type of symptom is evaluated currently, in the past 72 hours and in the past 3 months. Each of the four questions regarding frequency of symptoms is graded 0 (never) to 3 (constant), and each of the four severity questions is graded 0 (no symptoms) to 4 (intolerable symptoms). Scores are summed up and range from 0 to 28 [50].

Blink Rate, Incomplete Blink Rate (IBR), Interblink Interval (IBI), and Maximum Blink Interval (MBI)

Blink Rate

The patient should be observed for a period of time to calculate blink rate and time interval between blinks. The blink test can be an effective screening test for DED. Excessively low or high blink rates and intervals should be noted. The tear breakup during the blink interval is thought to result from a transient localized increase in osmolarity, which then stimulates the cornea nociceptors driving the blink reflex. The Optrex Dry Eye Blink test is a self-administered test with a reported sensitivity of 66% and a specificity of 88% in a group of 87 patients [47]. This has been used as a surrogate for detecting the loss of homeostasis as classified by TFOS DEWS II for Dry eye. Patients are instructed to look forward and record with a stopwatch the time when they felt discomfort following a blink. Averages of 3 measures per test was recommended. There was no need to remove contact lenses for this test. The blink test and NITBUT were not statistically different. There was also a significant negative correlation between the blink test and conjunctival lissamine staining [47, 51].

Incomplete Blink Rate

The LipiView device quantitates the number of incomplete blinks over a 20-s period and may provide important quantitative diagnostic information. It is also able to record both the maximum blink interval (MBI) and blink induction period (BIP), which have been correlated with DED [52, 53]. The BIP is the time from the TFBUT to the next blink and is calculated by subtracting the TFBUT from the MBI. The MBI is the number of seconds the eye can stay open without blinking, which is the sum of the TFBUT and the BIP (Fig. 4.4). The MBI has been shown to be highly correlated with the tear film breakup time (TFBUT) and is significantly shorter in patients with DED than normal. The MBI then provides important clinical information on the tear film function. The cutoff period for the MBI was 12.4 s with a positive predictive value of 76.9% and a negative predictive value of 59.5% [52, 53].

The interblink interval has also been shown to correlate with corneal sensation as corneal sensation also correlates with the tear film disruption [51, 54, 55].

External Facial Exam and Eyelid Position

External examination should begin with evaluation of the patient's periorbital and facial skin. Signs of rosacea including facial flushing and rhinophyma should be noted. The position of the eyelids, including ectropion, entropion, lid laxity (floppy eyelid syndrome), scleral show, and lagophthalmos should be noted.

Eyelid Laxity

Special consideration should be taken to evaluate for FES or palpebral hypermobility syndrome (PHS), which has a strong association with obstructive sleep apnea (OSA) and can play a role in meibomian gland dysfunction and ocular surface disease [16, 56–59].

Originally termed "floppy eyelid syndrome" by Culbertson in 1981 [60] describing eyelid laxity associated with chronic conjunctivitis in young obese men, this condition was been expanded by van

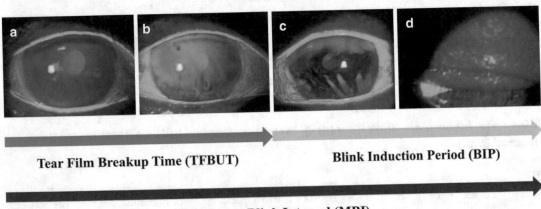

Fig. 4.4 TFBUT was the time interval between the last blink (**a**) and the appearance of the first dark spot on the cornea (**b**). MBI was the length of time that participants could keep the eye open before blinking (**a–d**). BIP was calculated by subtracting TFBUT from MBI (**c, d**). MBI: maximum blink interval; TFBUT tear film breakup time; BIP: blink interval period. (Inomata et al. [52]. Published under a CC BY 4.0 license)

den Bosch in 1994 [61] to include (1) lax eyelid condition (LEC), (a laxity of the eyelids in patients any age or weight not associated with conjunctivitis), (2) lax eyelid syndrome (LES) eyelid laxity in patient of any weight or sex associated with conjunctivitis, and then (3) FES as described by Culbertson. Elastin loss colocalized with MMP in the eyelids in pathology specimens of patients with FES has been reported [26]. The association of lax eyelids with MGD and MG dropout has been proposed [56, 58, 59]. The strong association of LES with obstructive sleep apnea (OSA) should also be recognized and patients referred for sleep study to alert patients at risk for multiple cardiovascular disease [62]. Tear MMP-9 has been elevated in patients with LES [56, 63, 64]. Abnormal corneal biomechanics (ocular response analyzer, ORA) has also been reported in patients with OSA perhaps associated with elevated MMP-9 in this patient population [64, 65].

OSA, which affects 25–30% adult men and 15–20% adult women in the United States, accounts for over $125 billion annually in the United States [66, 67]. Eighty percent of patients with OSA are undiagnosed. There may be a genetic association in Hispanic populations [68]. Several questionnaires including the STOP BANG questionnaire should be obtained to help identify patients at risk for OSA and a sleep study should be suggested if indicated.

Tear Osmolarity

Tear osmolarity has been shown to have the highest correlation with the most with disease severity out of the clinical dry eye disease tests in some studies, while others have shown significant variability in measurements [69]. Tear film osmolarity generally increased with greater disease burden. Patients with more severe disease tend to have higher tear osmolarity and larger differences between eyes. The tear osmolarity number and variability has been shown to decrease with treatment of the disease. Tear osmolarity of 308 mOsm/L or more or an interocular difference of greater than 8 mOSm/L has been accepted as the cutoff for a positive result.

Tear osmolarity can be measured with a TearLab Osmometer, which uses a strip at the tip of the TearLab pen that is placed in the lower tear meniscus for 2–3 s. The pen is then placed into the reader to provide a numerical measurement. No topical anesthetic is required for this measurement.

Meibography

There are a variety of techniques used to image the meibomian glands (Table 4.1) [29]. These include (1) meiboscopy, (2) meibography (contact and noncontact), and (3) confocal microscopy [34, 70]. Meibography describes the assessment of the meibomian gland anatomy.

Introduction to Meibography

Meibomian gland disease (MGD) is defined as a chronic, diffuse abnormality of the meibomian gland orifices that results in characteristic, visible, and quantifiable changes in meibomian gland quantity and structure [38]. MGD has been cited as a principal cause of posterior blepharitis, an inflammatory condition of the posterior lid margin [35]. This disease occurs more commonly in patients with rosacea, eczema, and atopy. These individuals commonly have lid margin abnormalities such as hyperemia, telangiectasias, and irregular lid margins [71]. Abnormal meibography has been shown in a variety of diseases including patients prior to BMT [31], chronic graft versus host disease [72], Stevens-Johnson syndrome [30, 32], sleep apnea [56], and a variety of ocular surface diseases [36, 53].

Defining Meiboscopy

Meiboscopy is a clinical examination technique used to assess the function of the central meibomian glands of the lower eyelid. This allows the clinician to obtain a gestalt of the meibomian gland involvement in the patient's blepharitis disease process. It is done by reflecting the central lower eyelid over a light probe, such as a muscle light, and examining the function, or lack thereof, of the central 8 meibomian glands with slit lamp illumination off.

Defining Meibography

The term "meibography" refers to the indirect visualization of the meibomian glands with imaging of the upper and lower eyelids. It was first described in 1977 by Tapie et al., whereas the actual term "meibography" was first coined by Mathers et al. in 1991 [40]. Now known as *contact meibography*, this technique involves the use of an infrared light probe to retroilluminate the everted eyelid from the skin and an ultraviolet light to illuminate and visualize meibomian gland presence and morphology. This requires an experienced examiner as it is difficult to perform and can cause significant patient discomfort. Additionally, contact meibography is a long and tedious process as the examiner is able to examine only the small area of retroilluminated eyelid at a time [24]. *Noncontact meibography* has become more widely used and is a faster, easier, more comfortable, and more complete exam to perform by allowing the photographer to obtain an image of all meibomian glands at once. It requires the use of a slit lamp microscope equipped with an infrared transmitting filter and an infrared charge coupled device camera system [24, 73]. This specialized device allows the clinician to capture both still and video images of meibomian gland structure (Figs. 4.5, 4.6, and 4.7).

Grading MGD Using Meibography

Standardized grading systems to define the findings observed in MGD have been critical in the diagnosis of this disease. The "meiboscore" and "meibograde" were terms defined by Arita et al. and Call et al., respectively, and are based on the appearance of meibomian glands on meibography imaging [24, 25, 74]. These grades can then be included with other objective findings of dry eye and tear film integrity to paint an objective picture of dry eye disease, which have defined treatment modalities [74].

The Meiboscore

The meiboscore was defined by Arita et al. in 2008 and employs the quantification of partial or complete meibomian gland dropout observed with meibography. In this system, individual eyelids are assigned a score based on the percentage of the total tarsal plate area that demonstrates gland dropout. A score out of three is then assigned for no dropout (grade 0), <33% dropout (grade 1), 33–66% dropout (grade 2), or >66% dropout (grade 3) [24].

The Meibograde

Coined by Call et al., the meibograde is a more detailed quantification of meibography image grading than the meiboscore [25]. It incorporates three objective descriptions of the meibomian glands into its scoring system: gland dropout, gland distortion, and gland shortening. These three are also ranked on a 0–3 scale, based on the percentage of the eyelid in which the changes are observed. The scores are added, and the individual eyelid is assigned a score out of nine. *Gland dropout* is defined as zones of the tarsal plate where glands should be but are not (Tables 4.1 and 4.2). Whichever grade the eyelid is given in the gland dropout category, the subsequent two scores necessarily must begin with that score. If an eyelid is given a grade of one on the gland dropout score, the grades in the subsequent two categories automatically begin at one. *Gland distortion* is defined as an abnormal gland-to-tarsus ratio, tortuosity of a gland, or the discordant pattern of the gland. Finally, *gland shortening* is graded based on percentage of eyelid demonstrating meibomian glands that do not extend from the eyelid margin to the opposite edge of the tarsal plate [25].

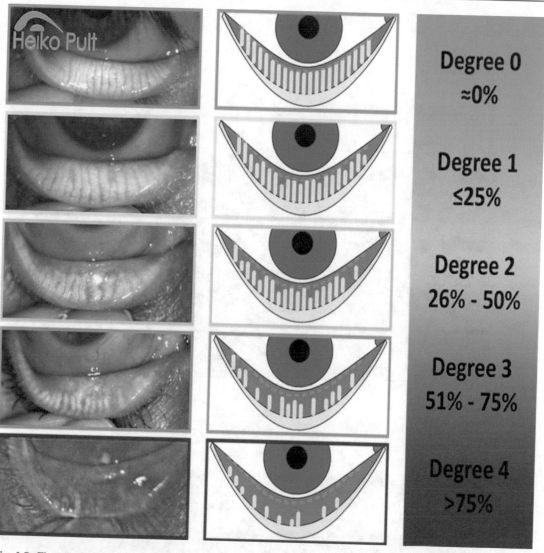

Fig. 4.5 Five-grade meiboscale to assess the severity of meibomian gland dropout. (Pult and Riede-Pult [74])

Anterior Eye Assessment

The lid margin and anterior eyelids should be examined thoroughly when assessing for blepharitis as these areas can exhibit a variety of pathologic changes. Lid margin rounding, hyperemia, increased vascularization, and hyperkeratinization are common [38]. These changes are exhibited by the blepharitis associated with rosacea [23]. A close assessment for *Demodex* infestation should be undertaken in the anterior eyelid, especially the lash follicles when anterior blepharitis is suspected [16]. *Demodex* infections are implicated in recurrent chalaza, which can also lead to DED [75].

A thorough anterior assessment of the eye in blepharitis is not complete without examination of the meibomian gland orifices and their relationship to the mucocutaneous junction. Normally, the meibomian gland orifices are located anterior to the mucocutaneous junction. With cicatricial changes, the

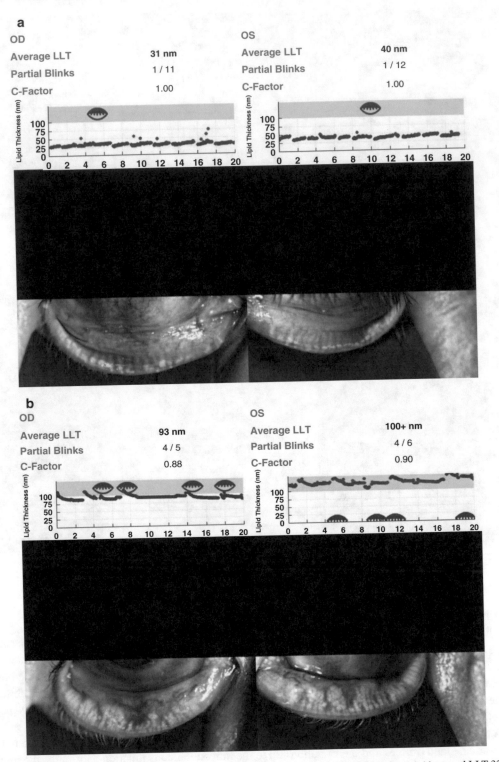

Fig. 4.6 LipiView images of meibography and lipid layer thickness (LLT) and partial blinks. (**a**) Abnormal LLT 32 nm OD and 40 nm OS with normal partial blink rate (1/11 OD and 1/12 OS with severe gland loss on meibography. (**b**) Normal LLT 93 nm OD and 100 + nm OS with abnormal partial blink rate 4/5 OD and 4/6 OS with moderate gland loss on meibography. (Reference: Courtesy of Charles Bouchard, MD)

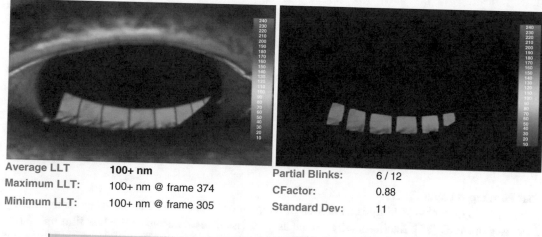

Average LLT	100+ nm	Partial Blinks:	6 / 12
Maximum LLT:	100+ nm @ frame 374	CFactor:	0.88
Minimum LLT:	100+ nm @ frame 305	Standard Dev:	11

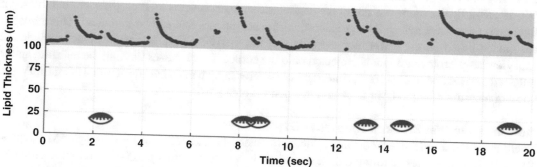

Fig. 4.7 LipiView images of tear interferometry and graphic representation of the lipid layer thickness (LLT) and partial blinks. With normal LLT 100+ nm with multiple partial blinks (6/12). (Reference: Courtesy of Charles Bouchard, MD)

mucocutaneous junction moves anteriorly, and the meibomian gland orifices move posteriorly onto the conjunctiva. These changes can be appreciated on an anterior eye examination [25, 37, 38].

Meibomian gland orifices show significant changes in blepharitis. Initially, capping of these orifices occurs as they undergo keratinization. This eventually develops into meibomian gland plugging and dropout. This process is a significant contributor to the evaporative aspect of DED that develops as a result of blepharitis [75].

The diagnosis of blepharitis and MGD can be characterized based on the quality and quantity of the material secreted by the meibomian glands. Hyposecretory MGD occurs when there is primary dysfunction of the glands and obstructive MGD involves a blockage of the meibomian gland orifices, leading to under-secretion from otherwise normal meibomian glands [2]. The meibum quality will appear clear or slightly cloudy in normal states versus the cloudy, granular, or inspissated quality of meibum secretion in MGD. This quality is best assessed on examination with gentle external pressure on the lower eyelid [37].

Tear Film Assessment

Structure

The tear film serves to protect the ocular surface and facilitates the spreading of the three tear components to provide optimal visual acuity [12]. The outer lipid layer is nonpolar and is made up of cholesterol and wax and cholesterol esters. The inner polar phospholipid layer contains intercalated proteins. The middle aqueous layer contains proteins, salts, and mucins (MUC5AC). The inner glycocalyx contains transmembrane glycoproteins and mucins (MUC 1, MUC 4, MUC 16). Tear film stability and composition will then determine the tear film breakup time (TFBUT), and lipid layer determined by interferometry inflammatory components can also be detected (i.e., MMP-9 (InflammaDry) [72, 76].

Lipid Layer Appearance (LLA)

The appearance of the lipid layer can be grossly assessed as having an open meshwork or a tight meshwork. The flow can be assessed, and the pattern can be structured or amorphous.

Tear Film Lipid Layer (TFLL)

The tear lipid thickness stability is a function of temperature and composition. This cycle of stability decreases in MGD [77]. Interferometry can be used to visualize and evaluate the tear film lipid layer [17, 18, 78, 79]. Tearscope was one of the first interferometers developed. It projects white fluorescent light onto the cornea, which then produces interference images that can be evaluated. These images are graded based on the uniformity and colors of the lipid film [23]. Newer machines include the LipiView interferometer. Light is projected onto the cornea, which passes through the tear film and is reflected into a camera. This creates interference patterns known as an interferogram. Using LipiView, one can measure the lipid layer thickness in a defined area [78].

Non-invasive Tear Breakup Time (NITBUT)

There are several objective automated systems to detect the TFBUT. The Keratograph 5M (Oculus, Wetzlar, Germany) uses an infrared light system to detect the first disruption of a projected mire pattern reflected from the corneal surface during the period of non-blinking [80]. An average of 3 "breakup time" measurements is determined. The time is calculated from the time interval from upstroke of blink to initial distortion. This method eliminates the disturbance from instillation of fluorescein and eliminates tactile reflex tearing. Breakup time measurements are generally longer using the NIBUT compared with the FBUT measurements, possibly a result of the destabilizing effect of the fluorescein. The sensitivity of 82% and sensitivity of 86% has been reported [79, 80]. Normal results for NITBUT have ranged from 40 to 60 s with abnormal measurement of less than 10 s. For the FBUT, the normal have been 10–345 s with an abnormal cutoff of <5 s [80].

Tear Meniscus Height (TMH)

The TMH can be measured by a variety of techniques and has been correlated with meibomian gland dysfunction [37, 79]. Classically, TMH is measured clinically via the instillation of fluorescein dye into the eye and evaluation of the height of the tear lake that accumulates between the lower eyelid and the globe. The emergence of new imaging techniques has allowed the clinician to measure TMH in a more non-invasive manner. It also eliminates the need for instilling drops in the patient's eyes prior to evaluating the tear meniscus height, an aspect of the exam that can skew results. Imaging devices such as the Keratograph 5M and LipiView have allowed the examiner to obtain more accurate measurements of TMH with the tear film in its more natural state [34, 79].

Tear Volume Testing

Schirmer Testing

Schirmer testing can be performed as a measure of aqueous tear production. For the Schirmer I test (without anesthesia), the strip of filter paper is folded at the notch and placed in the inferior fornix with the strip folded over the lateral lower lid margin. The patient is instructed to blink normally. The wetting of the strip is measured after 5 min. Variable diagnostic cutoff numbers have been suggested from <5 mm/5 min to <10 mm/5 min [3, 29, 75].

Schirmer without anesthesia with eyes closed can be used to distinguish between ADDE and EDE. A cutoff <5.5 mm at 5 min has a sensitivity of 85% and a specificity of 83%. There is generally a good correlation between MGD, Schirmer, Fluorescein staining but a poor correlation between Schirmer and dry eye symptoms [3, 12].

Phenol Red Testing

In this technique, a 70-mm long cotton thread impregnated with phenol red dye is used to collect the tears. This is pH sensitive and changed from yellow to red when exposed to tears. One eye is used to measure the volume and a 3-mm portion of the thread is placed in the lower outer third of the lid for 15 s. The patient may blink normally, and volume is determined from the length of the dye change [29].

Meibomian Gland Assessment

Overview

Meibomian gland disease (MGD) defined by the International Workshop on MGD as "is a chronic, diffuse abnormality of the meibomian glands, commonly characterized by terminal duct obstruction and/or qualitative/quantitative changes in the glandular secretion. This may result in alteration of the tear film, symptoms of eye irritation, clinically apparent inflammation and ocular surface disease" [29].

The two types of MGD are (1) low delivery states (most common) and (2) high delivery states. Low delivery, obstructive MGD results in a reduced meibum to the eyelid margin and tear film lipid layer leading to tear film instability, increased evaporation, tear hyperosmolarity, evaporative dry eye, and ocular surface inflammation and damage [81] (Fig. 4.1).

Meibomian Gland Expressibility (MGE)

MG expressibility is different from secretory activity and there are several published grading scales.

MG expressibility can be assessed using the Korb MG evaluator with a constant pressure for 10–15 s to the lower central 8 meibomian glands (TearScience, Morrisville, NC, USA) [37] (Fig. 4.2). The reported meibomian glands yielding liquid secretion (MGYLS) Score is then determined for the central 8/24 glands. Only some of the glands secrete at a time with the nasal being greater than middle greater than temporal glands. The grading scales are to distinguish between normal and abnormal with the expression not a measure of secretory activity. Table 4.2 illustrates other methods for evaluating MG expressibility with the specific grading scales [82].

Meibum Quality (MQ)

This was graded according to the scale listed below determined from the meibum expressed by the Korb evaluator [37]. This is graded on a 0–4 scale for each gland from clear fluid like (0) to thick like toothpaste (3) to obstructed without meibum expressed (4). The sum of the scores of the glands is then recorded. ($8 \times 3 = 24$ total).

Corneal Integrity Assessment

Ocular Surface Staining: Corneal and Conjunctival

Abnormal ocular surface staining, including corneal, conjunctival, and lid margin, can suggest ocular surface disease although not diagnostic [23]. Fluorescein dye, Rose Bengal, and Lissamine green are the commonly used dyes in the clinic. Fluorescein staining of epithelium occurs when the epithelial cells have lost their cell tight junctions or develop a defective glycocalyx [47].

Rose Bengal staining occurs where epithelial cells have lost their mucin or glycocalyx protective barrier. It also stains dead or degenerated epithelial cells. Rose Bengal tends to be irritating to the ocular surface and can induce reflex tearing. Therefore, its application should take place after assessment of tear film integrity and tear meniscus height.

Lissamine green stains epithelial cells that have damaged cell membranes, regardless of whether or not mucin is present. Lissamine green is better tolerated than Rose Bengal and therefore has become the preferred method for evaluation of patients with OSD. Recent reports of mixtures of several dyes show promise in staining the cornea and conjunctiva with a single drop [47].

There are several grading scales that have been developed to standardize the degree of ocular surface abnormality [29]. The van Bijsterveld grading system documents Rose Bengal epithelial staining using a scale of 0–3 on the cornea and two exposed areas of conjunctiva for a total score of 0–9. One drop of 1% Rose Bengal is used. The cutoff for normal is a score of greater than or equal to 3.5.

The Oxford Grading System grades ocular surface staining of the cornea and medial and lateral conjunctival segments using a score of 0–5 per zone for a total of 15.

The NEI/Industry scoring system uses a similar quadrant staining of the ocular surface. Tit uses 5 corneal and 2 × 3 conjunctival zones with a grade of 0–3 per zone. Fluorescein or Rose Bengal can be used.

Invasive Fluorescein Tear Film Breakup Time (IFBUT)

Invasive fluorescein tear breakup (IFBUT) time can be performed using several techniques. The most accurate is to instill 2 microliters of fluorescein into the inferior fornix/bulbar conjunctiva and measure the time to first break in tear film after a complete blink. Using the yellow barrier filter and the slit lamp at full height and 4 mm wide, the time from the upstroke of the last blink to the first breakup spot is recorded. The median value of 3 measurements is then recorded. The lower BUT between the two eyes should be the value considered for diagnosis. Alternatively, a fluorescein-impregnated strip is wetted with saline. The lack of control over volume of saline makes this unreliable. Measurement reliability increased with 2 ul or less of 5% solution. There seems to be no agreement on whether the strip should be shaken and where to apply the fluorescein, superiorly, inferiorly on the bulbar conjunctiva or tear meniscus. The cutoff often used as abnormal for this subjective measurement is less than 10 s for the strip and <5 s for 2 ul with a micropipette [47].

Lid Wiper and Bulbar Conjunctival Integrity Assessment

Lissamine green 10 ul volume is used to stain the upper lid using the Korb grading scale (0–3) measuring the horizontal length and sagittal height of the lid wiper. The bulbar conjunctival staining is determined from the Oxford grading scale. This grading scale uses a series of panels labeled A-E in order of increasing severity with representative images of staining patterns seen in ocular surface disease. The amount of staining increases by 0.5 of the log of the number of dots between panels B and E [83].

Inflammatory Mediators

MMP-9 (InflammaDry)

Matrix metalloproteinases are proteins found in the tear film in patients with dry eye disease. They are enzymes that can disrupt the ocular surface barrier. MMPs are secreted as inactive proenzymes and are activated by cleavage. InflammaDry is a point-of-care test, which measures levels of MMP-9 in the tear film. Value greater than 40 ng/ml is considered positive and a nonspecific indicator of ocular surface disease [75, 76].

Conclusion

Blepharitis, in particular meibomian gland dysfunction, is a complex disease process. Ocular surface health involves the delicate interaction between mechanical eyelid function, a chemically balanced tear film composition, adequate tear film integrity, and a healthy microbial micro-environment. As with any similarly complex disease process, the dysfunction of any one of these factors can result in a downward spiral of progressive ocular surface disease that is often difficult to eradicate. Often, patients present with improper functioning of many of these elements, making their diagnosis and treatment more difficult. Today's clinician must employ a multifaceted approach to diagnostic evaluation, grading of severity, and deployment of appropriate treatment plans. Diagnostic evaluation often includes history taking, patient examination, diagnostic testing, and photographic evaluation. Primary research and collaborative efforts in identifying this disease has led to innovative grading tools and scales that allow the clinician to evaluate one patient against another as well as a single patient's response to intervention. These diagnostic tools have made today's ophthalmologist more effective at treating blepharitis and, most importantly, improving their patient's sight and quality of life.

Compliance with Ethical Requirements   Roshni Vasaiwala, MD, Clayton Kirm, MD, and Charles Bouchard declare that they have no conflict of interest. No human or animal studies were carried out by the authors for this chapter.

References

1. Nelson JD, Shimazaki J, Benitez-del-Castillo JM, Craig JP, McCulley JP, Den S, et al. The international workshop on meibomian gland dysfunction: report of the definition and classification subcommittee. Invest Ophthalmol Vis Sci. 2011;52(4):1930–7.
2. Nichols KK, Foulks GN, Bron AJ, Glasgow BJ, Dogru M, Tsubota K, et al. The international workshop on meibomian gland dysfunction: executive summary. Invest Ophthalmol Vis Sci. 2011;52(4):1922–9.
3. Craig JP, Nelson JD, Azar DT, Belmonte C, Bron AJ, Chauhan SK, et al. TFOS DEWS II report executive summary. Ocul Surf. 2017;15(4):802–12.
4. Tsubota K, Yokoi N, Shimazaki J, Watanabe H, Dogru M, Yamada M, et al. New perspectives on dry eye definition and diagnosis: a consensus report by the Asia Dry Eye Society. Ocul Surf. 2017;15(1):65–76.
5. Yeotikar NS, Zhu H, Markoulli M, Nichols KK, Naduvilath T, Papas EB. Functional and morphologic changes of meibomian glands in an asymptomatic adult population. Invest Ophthalmol Vis Sci. 2016;57(10):3996–4007.
6. Schaumberg DA, Nichols JJ, Papas EB, Tong L, Uchino M, Nichols KK. The international workshop on meibomian gland dysfunction: report of the subcommittee on the epidemiology of, and associated risk factors for, MGD. Invest Ophthalmol Vis Sci. 2011;52(4):1994–2005.
7. Nichols KK. The international workshop on meibomian gland dysfunction: introduction. Invest Ophthalmol Vis Sci. 2011;52(4):1917–21.
8. Gilbard JP. Dry eye, blepharitis and chronic eye irritation: divide and conquer. J Ophthalmic Nurs Technol. 1999;18(3):109–15.
9. McCulley JP, Dougherty JM, Deneau DG. Classification of chronic blepharitis. Ophthalmology. 1982;89(10):1173–80.
10. Liu J, Sheha H, Tseng SC. Pathogenic role of Demodex mites in blepharitis. Curr Opin Allergy Clin Immunol. 2010;10(5):505–10.
11. Wolf R, Ophir J, Avigad J, Lengy J, Krakowski A. The hair follicle mites (Demodex spp.). Could they be vectors of pathogenic microorganisms? Acta Derm Venereol. 1988;68(6):535–7.
12. Craig JP, Nichols KK, Akpek EK, Caffery B, Dua HS, Joo CK, et al. TFOS DEWS II definition and classification report. Ocul Surf. 2017;15(3):276–83.
13. Knop E, Knop N, Millar T, Obata H, Sullivan DA. The international workshop on meibomian gland dysfunction: report of the subcommittee on anatomy, physiology, and pathophysiology of the meibomian gland. Invest Ophthalmol Vis Sci. 2011;52(4):1938–78.
14. Wu H, Wang Y, Dong N, Yang F, Lin Z, Shang X, et al. Meibomian gland dysfunction determines the severity of the dry eye conditions in visual display terminal workers. PLoS One. 2014;9(8):e105575.
15. Zhang X, Jeyalatha MV, Qu Y, He X, Ou S, Bu J, et al. Dry eye management: targeting the ocular surface microenvironment. Int J Mol Sci. 2017;18(7):1398.

16. Liu DT, Di Pascuale MA, Sawai J, Gao YY, Tseng SC. Tear film dynamics in floppy eyelid syndrome. Invest Ophthalmol Vis Sci. 2005;46(4):1188–94.

17. Kim JS, Lee H, Choi S, Kim EK, Seo KY, Kim TI. Assessment of the tear film lipid layer thickness after cataract surgery. Semin Ophthalmol. 2018;33(2):231–6.

18. Jung JW, Park SY, Kim JS, Kim EK, Seo KY, Kim TI. Analysis of factors associated with the tear film lipid layer thickness in normal eyes and patients with dry eye syndrome. Invest Ophthalmol Vis Sci. 2016;57(10):4076–83.

19. Hwang J-H, Lee J-H & Chung S-H. Comparison of Meibomian Gland Imaging Findings and Lipid Layer Thickness between Primary Sjögren Syndrome and Non-Sjögren Syndrome Dry Eyes, Ocular Immunology and Inflammation. 2020;28(2):182–87, https://doi.org/10.1080/09273948.2018.1562557.

20. Shtein RM, Shen JF, Kuo AN, Hammersmith KM, Li JY, Weikert MP. Autologous serum-based eye drops for treatment of ocular surface disease: a report by the American Academy of Ophthalmology. Ophthalmology. 2020;127(1):128–33.

21. Mizoguchi S, Iwanishi H, Arita R, Shirai K, Sumioka T, Kokado M, et al. Ocular surface inflammation impairs structure and function of meibomian gland. Exp Eye Res. 2017;163:78–84.

22. Randon M, Aragno V, Abbas R, Liang H, Labbe A, Baudouin C. In vivo confocal microscopy classification in the diagnosis of meibomian gland dysfunction. Eye (Lond). 2019;33(5):754–60.

23. Geerling G, Baudouin C, Aragona P, Rolando M, Boboridis KG, Benitez-Del-Castillo JM, et al. Emerging strategies for the diagnosis and treatment of meibomian gland dysfunction: proceedings of the OCEAN group meeting. Ocul Surf. 2017;15(2):179–92.

24. Arita R, Itoh K, Inoue K, Amano S. Noncontact infrared meibography to document age-related changes of the meibomian glands in a normal population. Ophthalmology. 2008;115(5):911–5.

25. Call CB, Wise RJ, Hansen MR, Carter KD, Allen RC. In vivo examination of meibomian gland morphology in patients with facial nerve palsy using infrared meibography. Ophthalmic Plast Reconstr Surg. 2012;28(6):396–400.

26. Gonnering RS, Sonneland PR. Meibomian gland dysfunction in floppy eyelid syndrome. Ophthalmic Plast Reconstr Surg. 1987;3(2):99–103.

27. Bergeron CM, Moe KS. The evaluation and treatment of lower eyelid paralysis. Facial Plast Surg. 2008;24(2):231–41.

28. Liang L, Liu Y, Ding X, Ke H, Chen C, Tseng SCG. Significant correlation between meibomian gland dysfunction and keratitis in young patients with Demodex brevis infestation. Br J Ophthalmol. 2018;102(8):1098–102.

29. Tomlinson A, Bron AJ, Korb DR, Amano S, Paugh JR, Pearce EI, et al. The international workshop on meibomian gland dysfunction: report of the diagnosis subcommittee. Invest Ophthalmol Vis Sci. 2011;52(4):2006–49.

30. Shrestha T, Moon HS, Choi W, Yoon HJ, Ji YS, Ueta M, et al. Characteristics of meibomian gland dysfunction in patients with Stevens-Johnson syndrome. Medicine (Baltimore). 2019;98(26):e16155.

31. Giannaccare G, Bonifazi F, Sebastiani S, Sessa M, Pellegrini M, Arpinati M, et al. Meibomian gland dropout in hematological patients before hematopoietic stem cell transplantation. Cornea. 2018;37(10):1264–9.

32. Lekhanont K, Jongkhajornpong P, Sontichai V, Anothaisintawee T, Nijvipakul S. Evaluating dry eye and meibomian gland dysfunction with meibography in patients with Stevens-Johnson syndrome. Cornea. 2019;38(12):1489–94.

33. Mathers WD, Daley T, Verdick R. Video imaging of the meibomian gland. Arch Ophthalmol. 1994;112(4):448–9.

34. Wong S, Srinivasan S, Murphy PJ, Jones L. Comparison of meibomian gland dropout using two infrared imaging devices. Cont Lens Anterior Eye. 2019;42(3):311–7.

35. McCann LC, Tomlinson A, Pearce EI, Diaper C. Tear and meibomian gland function in blepharitis and normals. Eye Contact Lens. 2009;35(4):203–8.

36. Suzuki T, Morishige N, Arita R, Koh S, Sakimoto T, Shirakawa R, et al. Morphological changes in the meibomian glands of patients with phlyctenular keratitis: a multicenter cross-sectional study. BMC Ophthalmol. 2016;16(1):178.

37. Korb DR, Blackie CA. Meibomian gland therapeutic expression: quantifying the applied pressure and the limitation of resulting pain. Eye Contact Lens. 2011;37(5):298–301.

38. Putnam CM. Diagnosis and management of blepharitis: an optometrist's perspective. Clin Optom (Auckl). 2016;8:71–8.

39. Pflugfelder SC. Antiinflammatory therapy for dry eye. Am J Ophthalmol. 2004;137(2):337–42.

40. Mathers WD, Shields WJ, Sachdev MS, Petroll WM, Jester JV. Meibomian gland dysfunction in chronic blepharitis. Cornea. 1991;10(4):277–85.

41. Shimazaki J, Sakata M, Tsubota K. Ocular surface changes and discomfort in patients with meibomian gland dysfunction. Arch Ophthalmol. 1995;113(10):1266–70.

42. de Paiva CS. Effects of aging in dry eye. Int Ophthalmol Clin. 2017;57(2):47–64.

43. Maruyama Y, Ikeda Y, Yokoi N, Mori K, Kato H, Ueno M, et al. Severe corneal disorders developed after brimonidine tartrate ophthalmic solution use. Cornea. 2017;36(12):1567–9.

44. Kato M, Nitta K, Kano Y, Yamada M, Ishii N, Hashimoto T, et al. Case of phenylephrine hydrochloride-induced periorbital contact dermatitis with fulminant keratoconjunctivitis causing pseudomembrane formation. J Dermatol. 2018;45(2):e27–e8.

45. Wang S, Zhao H, Huang C, Li Z, Li W, Zhang X, et al. Impact of chronic smoking on meibomian gland dysfunction. PLoS One. 2016;11(12):e0168763.

46. Dougherty BE, Nichols JJ, Nichols KK. Rasch analysis of the ocular surface disease index (OSDI). Invest Ophthalmol Vis Sci. 2011;52(12):8630–5.

47. Wolffsohn JS, Craig JP, Vidal-Rohr M, Huarte ST, Ah Kit L, Wang M. Blink test enhances ability to screen for dry eye disease. Cont Lens Anterior Eye. 2018;41(5):421–5.

48. Schiffman RM, Christianson MD, Jacobsen G, Hirsch JD, Reis BL. Reliability and validity of the ocular surface disease index. Arch Ophthalmol. 2000;118(5):615–21.

49. Chalmers RL, Begley CG, Caffery B. Validation of the 5-item dry eye questionnaire (DEQ-5): discrimination across self-assessed severity and aqueous tear deficient dry eye diagnoses. Cont Lens Anterior Eye. 2010;33(2):55–60.

50. Ngo W, Situ P, Keir N, Korb D, Blackie C, Simpson T. Psychometric properties and validation of the standard patient evaluation of eye dryness questionnaire. Cornea. 2013;32(9):1204–10.

51. Jie Y, Sella R, Feng J, Gomez ML, Afshari NA. Evaluation of incomplete blinking as a measurement of dry eye disease. Ocul Surf. 2019;17(3):440–6.

52. Inomata T, Iwagami M, Hiratsuka Y, Fujimoto K, Okumura Y, Shiang T, et al. Maximum blink interval is associated with tear film breakup time: a new simple, screening test for dry eye disease. Sci Rep. 2018;8(1):13443.

53. Park J, Kim J, Lee H, Park M, Baek S. Functional and structural evaluation of the meibomian gland using a LipiView interferometer in thyroid eye disease. Can J Ophthalmol. 2018;53(4):373–9.

54. Varikooty J, Simpson TL. The interblink interval I: the relationship between sensation intensity and tear film disruption. Invest Ophthalmol Vis Sci. 2009;50(3):1087–92.

55. Johnston PR, Rodriguez J, Lane KJ, Ousler G, Abelson MB. The interblink interval in normal and dry eye subjects. Clin Ophthalmol. 2013;7:253–9.

56. Karaca I, Yagci A, Palamar M, Tasbakan MS, Basoglu OK. Ocular surface assessment and morphological alterations in meibomian glands with meibography in obstructive sleep apnea syndrome. Ocul Surf. 2019;17(4):771–6.

57. Giannaccare G, Bernabei F, Pellegrini M, Arpinati M, Bonifazi F, Sessa M, et al. Eyelid metrics assessment in patients with chronic ocular graft versus-host disease. Ocul Surf. 2019;17(1):98–103.

58. Chhadva P, McClellan AL, Alabiad CR, Feuer WJ, Batawi H, Galor A. Impact of eyelid laxity on symptoms and signs of dry eye disease. Cornea. 2016;35(4):531–5.

59. Mastrota KM. Impact of floppy eyelid syndrome in ocular surface and dry eye disease. Optom Vis Sci. 2008;85(9):814–6.

60. Culbertson WW, Ostler HB. The floppy eyelid syndrome. Am J Ophthalmol. 1981;92(4):568–75.

61. van den Bosch WA, Lemij HG. The lax eyelid syndrome. Br J Ophthalmol. 1994;78(9):666–70.

62. Javaheri S, Barbe F, Campos-Rodriguez F, Dempsey JA, Khayat R, Javaheri S, et al. Sleep apnea: types, mechanisms, and clinical cardiovascular consequences. J Am Coll Cardiol. 2017;69(7):841–58.

63. Sward M, Kirk C, Kumar S, Nasir N, Adams W, Bouchard C. Lax eyelid syndrome (LES), obstructive sleep apnea (OSA), and ocular surface inflammation. Ocul Surf. 2018;16(3):331–6.

64. Chotikavanich S, de Paiva CS, Li de Q, Chen JJ, Bian F, Farley WJ, et al. Production and activity of matrix metalloproteinase-9 on the ocular surface increase in dysfunctional tear syndrome. Invest Ophthalmol Vis Sci. 2009;50(7):3203–9.

65. Nadarajah S, Samsudin A, Ramli N, Tan CT, Mimiwati Z. Corneal hysteresis is reduced in obstructive sleep apnea syndrome. Optom Vis Sci. 2017;94(10):981–5.

66. Young T, Evans L, Finn L, Palta M. Estimation of the clinically diagnosed proportion of sleep apnea syndrome in middle-aged men and women. Sleep. 1997;20(9):705–6.

67. Young T, Palta M, Dempsey J, Skatrud J, Weber S, Badr S. The occurrence of sleep-disordered breathing among middle-aged adults. N Engl J Med. 1993;328(17):1230–5.

68. Cade BE, Chen H, Stilp AM, Gleason KJ, Sofer T, Ancoli-Israel S, et al. Genetic associations with obstructive sleep apnea traits in Hispanic/Latino Americans. Am J Respir Crit Care Med. 2016;194(7):886–97.

69. Sullivan BD, Whitmer D, Nichols KK, Tomlinson A, Foulks GN, Geerling G, et al. An objective approach to dry eye disease severity. Invest Ophthalmol Vis Sci. 2010;51(12):6125–30.

70. Wise RJ, Sobel RK, Allen RC. Meibography: a review of techniques and technologies. Saudi J Ophthalmol. 2012;26(4):349–56.

71. AlDarrab A, Alrajeh M, Alsuhaibani AH. Meibography for eyes with posterior blepharitis. Saudi J Ophthalmol. 2017;31(3).131–4.

72. Ban Y, Ogawa Y, Goto E, Uchino M, Terauchi N, Seki M, et al. Tear function and lipid layer alterations in dry eye patients with chronic graft-vs-host disease. Eye (Lond). 2009;23(1):202–8.

73. Mohamed Mostafa E, Abdellah MM, Elhawary AM, Mounir A. Noncontact meibography in patients with keratoconus. J Ophthalmol. 2019;2019:2965872.

74. Pult H, Riede-Pult B. Comparison of subjective grading and objective assessment in meibography. Cont Lens Anterior Eye. 2013;36(1):22–7.

75. Wolffsohn JS, Arita R, Chalmers R, Djalilian A, Dogru M, Dumbleton K, et al. TFOS DEWS II diagnostic methodology report. Ocul Surf. 2017;15(3):539–74.
76. Sambursky R, Davitt WF 3rd, Latkany R, Tauber S, Starr C, Friedberg M, et al. Sensitivity and specificity of a point-of-care matrix metalloproteinase 9 immunoassay for diagnosing inflammation related to dry eye. JAMA Ophthalmol. 2013;131(1):24–8.
77. Milner MS, Beckman KA, Luchs JI, Allen QB, Awdeh RM, Berdahl J, et al. Dysfunctional tear syndrome: dry eye disease and associated tear film disorders – new strategies for diagnosis and treatment. Curr Opin Ophthalmol. 2017;27(Suppl 1):3–47.
78. Sang X, Li Y, Yang L, Liu JH, Wang XR, Li CY, et al. Lipid layer thickness and tear meniscus height measurements for the differential diagnosis of evaporative dry eye subtypes. Int J Ophthalmol. 2018;11(9):1496–502.
79. Tong L, Teng LS. Review of literature on measurements of non-invasive break up times, lipid morphology and tear meniscal height using commercially available hand-held instruments. Curr Eye Res. 2018;43(5):567–75.
80. Tian L, Qu JH, Zhang XY, Sun XG. Repeatability and reproducibility of noninvasive keratograph 5M measurements in patients with dry eye disease. J Ophthalmol. 2016;2016:8013621.
81. Yoo YS, Na KS, Byun YS, Shin JG, Lee BH, Yoon G, et al. Examination of gland dropout detected on infrared meibography by using optical coherence tomography meibography. Ocul Surf. 2017;15(1):130–8. e1
82. Engel LA, Wittig S, Bock F, Sauerbier L, Scheid C, Holtick U, et al. Meibography and meibomian gland measurements in ocular graft-versus-host disease. Bone Marrow Transplant. 2015;50(7):961–7.
83. Bron AJ, de Paiva CS, Chauhan SK, Bonini S, Gabison EE, Jain S, et al. TFOS DEWS II pathophysiology report. Ocul Surf. 2017;15(3):438–510.
84. Shimazaki J, Sakata M, Tsubota K. Ocular surface changes and discomfort in patients with meibomian gland dysfunction. Arch Ophthalmol. 1995;113(10):1266–70.
85. Henriquez AS and Korb DR. Meibomian glands and contact lens wear. Journal of Ophthalmology. 1981;65: 108–111.
86. Arita R, Suehiro J, Haraguchi T, et al. Objective image analysis of the meibomian gland area. Br J Ophthalmol. 2014;98:746.

Sebaceous Carcinoma: Masquerade Syndrome

Johnathan Jeffers, Megan Silas, and Hassan Shah

Introduction

Sebaceous carcinoma is a malignant neoplasm arising from the sebaceous glands [1–3]. First identified in 1891 by Allaire, sebaceous carcinoma rose to clinical prominence following publication of a series of 21 meibomian gland tumors by Stratsmaa in 1956 [3, 4]. Sebaceous carcinoma has historically been referred to by various names including meibomian gland carcinoma [4, 5], sebaceous gland carcinoma [6, 7], and sebaceous cell carcinoma [8]. Consensus today has settled on sebaceous carcinoma as the eponym for malignancy arising from the sebaceous glands [1, 2]. The neoplasm is most often found in the periocular region where sebaceous glands are numerous. Sebaceous glands are found most prominently in the tarsus, as the meibomian glands, followed by the cilia [Zeiss glands], eyebrow, and the caruncle. Extraocular sites include the parotid and submandibular glands, as well as sebaceous glands of the skin, especially in the head and neck region [3, 9].

Though relatively rare, sebaceous carcinoma is the second most common eyelid malignancy behind basal cell carcinoma [1]. The disease remains predominantly a malignancy of the elderly, though cases have been reported in the pediatric population [10].

Sebaceous carcinoma most often results from de novo mutations, resulting in a sporadic, non-heritable disease pattern. However, a heritable form of the disease, termed Muir-Torre syndrome (MTS) has been identified. MTS is a subtype of hereditary non-polyposis colorectal cancer syndrome (HNPCC), which is associated with the development of sebaceous tumors, keratoacanthomas, and visceral malignancies [11]. These clusters of malignancies are related to mutations in DNA mismatch repair proteins that result in microsatellite instability and a predisposition to genetic defects in replicating cells. Thus, in patients with newly diagnosed sebaceous carcinoma, it is important to obtain a thorough family history of malignancy to determine the possible need for further genetic testing and follow-up [2].

J. Jeffers
University of Chicago Pritzker School of Medicine, Chicago, IL, USA

M. Silas · H. Shah (✉)
University of Chicago Medical Center, Department of Ophthalmology and Visual Science, Chicago, IL, USA
e-mail: hshah1@bsd.uchicago.edu

© Springer Nature Switzerland AG 2021
A. V. Farooq, J. J. Reidy (eds.), *Blepharitis*, Essentials in Ophthalmology,
https://doi.org/10.1007/978-3-030-65040-7_5

Sebaceous carcinoma is often referred to as the great masquerader for its ability to mimic more prevalent and often benign eyelid disorders characterized by prominent inflammatory reactions such as blepharitis and chalazion. Sebaceous carcinoma can present as a subcutaneous nodule. However, presentation may be limited to discreet eyelid thickening. The disease's relatively low prevalence, combined with its ability to present in a multitude of ways, makes it a difficult disease to detect. As such, it requires an astute clinician to consistently include sebaceous carcinoma in the list of possible differential diagnoses in patients presenting with eyelid complaints [12, 13].

Primary management of sebaceous carcinoma consists of complete surgical resection. Secondary management may include topical chemotherapy, cryotherapy, and amniotic membrane grafting [1–3]. Map biopsies of the surrounding lid and conjunctiva are often necessary given the propensity of sebaceous carcinoma to undergo intraepithelial pagetoid spread [14]. Prognosis for sebaceous carcinoma depends primarily on the extent of invasion into surrounding tissues and structures, as well as the presence of distant metastases to regional lymph nodes or solid organs [7]. Increasing awareness of the disease may lead to early diagnosis and better outcomes for patients affected by the disease.

This chapter takes an in-depth look at ocular adnexal sebaceous carcinoma including its epidemiology, pathogenesis, origins, clinical presentation, differential diagnoses, histology, diagnosis, management strategies, and prognosis.

Epidemiology

In the United States, the incidence of sebaceous carcinoma has been estimated to be 0.11 per 100,000 people [11]. It represents approximately 1–5.5% of eyelid malignancies and is second behind basal cell carcinoma in terms of frequency [3]. Sebaceous carcinoma most frequently occurs on the eyelid (38.7%), but it is known to occur in any sebaceous gland containing tissues, primarily in the head and neck region [9]. It has been suggested that the incidence in the United States has been increasing, but this may possibly be a result of increased rates of detection [15].

Sebaceous carcinoma is a disease of the elderly, with an average age of onset of 73 years. Many reports have indicated a female predominance in development of the malignancy. However, a few recent studies have called into question this association and suggest a possible male predominance [9, 11]. Asian countries have the highest reported incidence of sebaceous carcinoma, with some studies finding rates ranging from as high as 7.9 to 10.2% of all eyelid malignancies [16, 17]. In the United States, whites are most affected by the disease (2.03 per 1,000,000) followed by Asian/Pacific Islanders (1.07 per 1,000,000) and blacks (0.48 per 1,000,000) [9].

Risk factors for sebaceous carcinoma include a history of radiation exposure, HPV infection, Muir-Torre syndrome, retinoblastoma, HIV infection, and systemic immunosuppression such as chronic steroid usage [1, 10, 11, 18, 19]. The role of the immune system in preventing tumor formation has been well studied, and immunosuppression remains a major risk factor for development of sebaceous carcinoma. Patients infected with HIV have an 8 times greater risk of developing sebaceous carcinoma than the general population [18]. Prior radiation exposure, especially to the ocular region, increases the risk of developing sebaceous carcinoma. Another risk factor, particularly in the pediatric population, includes a history of familial retinoblastoma. This association is likely confounded by the usage of radiation to treat initial occurrences of retinoblastoma. In one study, patients were found to develop sebaceous carcinoma on average 5–15 years following radiation exposure [10]. Finally, Muir-Torre syndrome (MTS) is an autosomal dominant condition caused by known mutations in DNA mismatch repair proteins including MLH1 and MSH2. MTS is associated with an increased risk of developing sebaceous tumors, including sebaceous carcinoma [11].

Pathogenesis

The pathogenesis of sebaceous carcinoma is not wholly understood [1, 2]. Muir-Torre syndrome has been implicated in familial forms of sebaceous carcinoma. The mutated DNA mismatch repair genes (*MLH1/MLH2*) discussed above result in microsatellite instability and subsequent hyper-mutability of cancer cells [2, 11]. However, sporadic forms of sebaceous carcinoma do not appear to share a similar pathogenesis to those associated with Muir-Torre syndrome. Various studies have pointed to a role of p53, the known tumor suppressor protein, in progression of sebaceous carcinoma. Other studies have identified infection by human papilloma virus (HPV) as a potential factor in promoting the development of the malignancy [20]. Researchers have examined p16 as a possible surrogate marker for periocular sebaceous carcinoma, given its known overexpression in extraocular sebaceous carcinoma. However, no association was found between expression of p16 and periocular sebaceous carcinomas [21].

Inactivation of the p53 tumor suppressor protein in cells infected by HPV has been well established in the development of mucosa-associated cancers, including cervical cancer. HPV acts by gaining entrance to epithelial cells and utilizing the cellular machinery to transcribe and translate oncogenic genes into proteins. One such oncogenic protein, E6, has been shown to work through binding and inactivating p53, leading to an increased proteasome-dependent degradation of the cell-cycle-modulating protein. Loss of this important protein thus leads to a decoupling of regular cellular checkpoints and results in unchecked cellular proliferation. Similarly, the HPV-associated oncogenic protein E7 is known to deactivate another tumor suppressor protein, pRB [20]. Thus, this viral-associated mechanism could provide a cellular pathway for the increased risk of developing sebaceous carcinoma seen in patients with familial retinoblastoma.

The mechanism of malignant conversion in non-HPV-associated sebaceous carcinomas differs from those associated with the virus. In fact, nuclear staining for p53 is increased, particularly in eyelid sebaceous carcinomas compared to more benign extraocular lesions [22]. Previous studies have noted an increased production of the mutated p53 tumor suppressor protein in sebaceous carcinoma, suggesting a possible role of p53 mutations in progression of the malignancy [23, 24]. In fact, common p53 mutations have been found in functional domains related to its action as a DNA-binding protein. An altered amino-acid structure leads to diminished molecular interactions with deoxyribonucleic acid and a subsequent decrease in p53's ability to act as a transcription factor. Thus, it appears that mutational inactivation of p53 promotes tumorigenesis, despite increased expression patterns in sebaceous carcinoma. Overexpression of p53 was also thought to correlate with more advanced or aggressive lesions [25]. However, recent evidence suggests otherwise, as different stages of sebaceous carcinomas do not show varied expression patterns of the mutant protein. Though p53 does appear to be implicated in sebaceous carcinoma, it may be more important in early carcinogenesis than in disease progression [23].

Clinical Presentation and Tissue Origin

Sebaceous carcinoma is known to mimic more benign diseases and has a variety of clinical presentations. This feature has earned the disease the title of "The Masquerade Syndrome" [1–3]. This section will examine the clinical presentation and tissue origin of the malignancy. It is important for clinicians, especially ophthalmologists, to be aware of the variety of presentations of sebaceous carcinoma. Delays in diagnosis can result in increased rates of metastasis and poorer outcomes. Given the possibility of the malignancy to be cured with complete surgical removal, early detection and diagnosis is key to proper management of the disease.

Ocular Adnexal Origin

Sebaceous carcinoma is most often found in the ocular adnexal region. Estimates for the percentage of sebaceous carcinomas occurring in the periorbital region range from 40% to 75% [9, 26]. The most common ocular sites in order of occurrence are the meibomian glands, glands of Zeiss, caruncle, eyebrow, and conjunctiva [1–3]. Finally, some malignancies are thought to stem from a multicentric origin of two or more of these discrete areas, though in many advanced cases the site of origin remains unknown [27].

Meibomian Glands

The meibomian glands represent the most common single site for development of ocular adnexal sebaceous carcinomas [27, 28]. The vast majority of sebaceous carcinomas occurring within the periocular region arise from the meibomian glands of the upper lid [27, 29]. Presentation of the malignancy can range from simple eyelid thickening, to a discrete, firm, and painless nodule. Patients can present with a subcutaneous nodule, which is often fixed to the tarsus [26]. Figure 5.1 shows sebaceous carcinoma of the upper eyelid. The nodules are often yellow in color, likely related to the high lipid content [1, 2, 29]. These lesions may be easily mistaken for a chalazion. Eyelid thickening can present a more challenging diagnosis for clinicians, as the thickening is often accompanied with an inflammatory reaction that can mimic blepharitis [12, 13]. As a result, management of sebaceous carcinoma that presents as diffuse thickening of the eyelid requires more extensive map biopsies to document the extent of invasion prior to any resection [14].

Glands of Zeiss

The glands of Zeiss, found associated with the eyelash hair follicles, are the second most common orbital sites for development of sebaceous carcinoma. Approximately 10% of orbital sebaceous carcinomas arise from these glands [29]. Similar to lesions developing in the meibomian glands, lesions originating from the glands of Zeiss may be mistaken for chalazia near the eyelid margin. One important sign that helps to assist in differentiating between a benign process such as chalazion, versus sebaceous carcinoma, is madarosis, or loss of cilia. As the malignancy invades the surround-

Fig. 5.1 Sebaceous carcinoma of the upper eyelid. (Knackstedt and Samie [30])

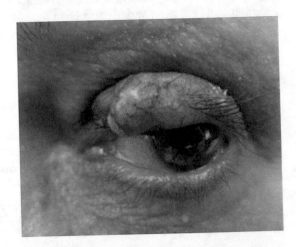

ing tissue, it often obliterates the surrounding hair follicles, leading to the loss of eyelashes along the lid margin [8]. Thus, a detailed slit-lamp exam can help guide the clinician in determining the proper diagnosis.

Caruncle

Sebaceous carcinoma of the caruncle is rare, representing only 3% of all periocular sebaceous carcinomas [29]. The caruncle contains fine lanugo type hair, which harbor sebaceous glands within their associated hair follicles. Sebaceous carcinoma in the caruncle often presents as a firm, painless nodule, but has also been seen to grow in a more verrucous or pedunculated type pattern [1].

Eyebrow

Sebaceous carcinoma may arise from the pilosebaceous units of the hair follicles of the eyebrow, though this presentation is rare [3, 30]. Often presenting as a firm nodule, the malignancy may progress to an ulcerated, painful brow lesion [31]. These tumors can also mimic sebaceous or epidermal inclusion cysts [32].

Conjunctiva

It has been disputed whether sebaceous carcinoma can arise directly from the conjunctiva. Various studies have suggested that the conjunctiva represents a primary area for development of the malignancy [1, 33]. However, it is generally thought that sebaceous carcinoma within the conjunctiva represents intraepithelial pagetoid spread from a primary lesion within the eyelid. Given the varied patterns in presentation of the malignancy, it may be initially difficult to detect the primary lesion, leading to a misappropriation of the conjunctiva as a site of development of sebaceous carcinoma [27]. Nonetheless, a detailed slit-lamp exam and map biopsies of the conjunctiva are often necessary to determine the presence of spread from the primary site, given the malignancy's predilection for invading the surrounding conjunctiva.

Extraocular Sites

The head and neck region encompasses most of the other sites implicated in the development of sebaceous carcinoma. These sites include the parotid and submandibular glands and skin of the head and neck. However, the disease can occur on the chest, abdomen, extremities, and genitalia [34]. It is believed that sun exposure represents an important causal role in development of sebaceous carcinoma, given the increased rates of development in sun-exposed areas of the head and neck. However, case reports of sebaceous carcinoma arising from the external genitalia suggest a more prominent role of HPV in development of the tumor [35]. These tumors can often mimic other dermatologic malignancies including squamous cell and basal cell carcinomas. Biopsy remains essential in differentiating between these malignancies and more benign processes [2]. Non-ocular adnexal sebaceous carcinoma presents similarly to adnexal forms of the malignancy in that it is often a firm nodule that eventually ulcerates in later stages of the disease. These sebaceous carcinomas are known to progress to ulceration more rapidly than periocular tumors, but both forms of the malignancy appear to have similar prognoses [36].

Fig. 5.2 Sebaceous carcinoma of lower eyelid margin presenting as chronic blepharitis. (Schmitz et al. [76])

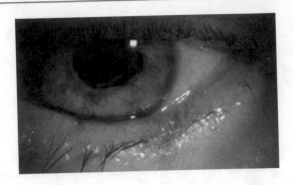

Differential Diagnosis

Lesions suggestive of sebaceous carcinoma should garner a broad differential resulting from the disease's ability to masquerade as various inflammatory and oncogenic processes [12]. The varied presentation pattern of sebaceous carcinoma from a small, discrete eyelid nodule to global eyelid inflammation and thickening of the tarsus requires an astute clinician for prompt diagnosis. Given the wide array of presentations and difficulty in distinguishing it from benign ocular tumors, tissue biopsy is required for definitive diagnosis [13]. This section examines some of the major diseases included in the differential for sebaceous carcinoma.

Blepharitis

Sebaceous carcinoma's tendency to present with diffuse involvement of the eyelid and subsequent inflammation often leads to its mischaracterization as blepharitis. There are several key features that can help distinguish sebaceous carcinoma from blepharitis including trichiasis, madarosis, and overt eyelid thickening [1, 3, 15]. Furthermore, blepharitis, including that resulting from demodex infection, often results in dandruff-like deposits, or collarettes, at the bases of the lashes [37]. Figure 5.2 shows sebaceous carcinoma masquerading as chronic blepharitis.

Chalazion

Chalazia present as eyelid nodules and most often result in intense inflammatory reactions accompanied by significant swelling, erythema, and pain. As discussed in the section on clinical presentation, the most common presentation of sebaceous carcinoma is a painless, round nodule on the upper eyelid. As such, sebaceous carcinoma can be easily misdiagnosed as a chalazion [1–3]. Chalazia often occur in young people, and do not require biopsy. However, any recurrent chalazion should undergo biopsy to rule out malignancy, especially in older individuals [38].

Conjunctivitis

Conjunctivitis often presents as a bilateral process, though unilateral disease is not uncommon. Sebaceous carcinoma is known to undergo pagetoid invasion of the surrounding corneal and conjunctival epithelium. The infiltration may include the bulbar, forniceal, and palpebral conjunctiva [39].

This invasion can lead to an inflammatory reaction and subsequent erythema within the conjunctiva and cornea that mimics conjunctivitis, making it difficult to properly diagnose [40]. In these cases, multiple biopsies may be required to determine the extent of invasion and to guide appropriate treatment for the disease [14].

Keratitis

The inflammatory reaction instigated by sebaceous carcinoma can also result in pannus formation overlying the cornea. These can be mistaken for simple pterygium. As the pagetoid spread continues from the conjunctival epithelium to the corneal epithelium, a picture of marginal keratitis may emerge [41]. The underlying inflammatory reaction can progress, resulting in peripheral ulcerative keratitis [42].

Superior Limbic Keratoconjunctivitis

Given the propensity for sebaceous carcinoma to arise in the upper eyelid, the local invasion and subsequent inflammation of the superior conjunctiva may mimic superior limbic keratoconjunctivitis [SLK]. The inflammatory disorder is characterized by papillary inflammation of the superior perilimbal, tarsal, and bulbar conjunctiva. As the malignancy spreads, sebaceous carcinoma may be mistaken for SLK. In fact, of all of the diseases sebaceous carcinoma mimics, SLK is one of the few that can also present as an inflammatory thickening of the superior eyelid. The chronicity of this disease and similar features of this disease may make subsequent recognition and treatment of sebaceous carcinoma difficult in those misdiagnosed with SLK [43].

Squamous Cell Carcinoma

In contrast to sebaceous carcinoma, which has a predilection for the upper eyelid, squamous cell carcinoma most often occurs on the lower lid. The malignancy also disproportionately affects older individuals, much like sebaceous carcinoma. Squamous cell carcinoma may also occur as a nodular or more papillomatous appearance. It usually presents as an indurated papule with an erythematous border, which frequently progresses to ulceration. Time to ulceration is generally much shorter in squamous cell carcinoma as compared to basal cell carcinoma and sebaceous carcinoma [44].

Basal Cell Carcinoma

Periocular basal cell carcinoma is most often found on the medial canthus and lower eyelid. Basal cell carcinoma is the most common orbital malignancy, representing 80–90% of periocular tumors. It is also the most common malignant tumor overall in humans. Despite its frequency, it is rarely known to metastasize until the late stages of the disease. However, periocular basal carcinoma causes high rates of morbidity given its tendency to invade the surrounding tissue. Similar to squamous cell carcinoma, basal cell carcinoma often begins as a small pearly nodule that eventually progresses to ulceration. Definitive differentiation from other malignancies, including sebaceous carcinoma, requires biopsy and histopathological diagnosis [45].

Melanoma

Ocular melanoma most often arises within the uveal tissues of the eye. However, the malignancy may also arise from the conjunctiva, eyelid, and surrounding orbital skin. Conjunctival melanoma presents as a pigmented lesion on the conjunctival surface that can be misdiagnosed as a benign nevus. Primary melanotic lesions of the eyelid are quite rare. However, eyelid lesions can represent foci of metastatic disease [46]. Interestingly, a previously excised melanotic lesion on the eyelid may recur as a non-pigmented lesion resembling sebaceous carcinoma [1]. Recurrent lesions may require exteneration because of the difficulty in detection and the high rates of metastasis [46].

Mucinous Eccrine Adenocarcinoma

Mucinous eccrine adenocarcinoma is a rare periocular tumor that typically presents as a solitary lesion that can be transilluminated due to its high mucin content. Its presentation is often variable, making it difficult to diagnose clinically. Though rates of metastasis remain low, recurrence rates approach roughly 50%, making mucinous eccrine adenocarcinoma difficult to treat effectively. Like sebaceous carcinoma, mucinous eccrine adenocarcinoma is a malignancy that commonly affects the elderly with an average age of onset in the low 60s [47].

Mucoepidermoid Carcinoma

Mucoepidermoid carcinoma is an extremely rare epithelial neoplasm [48]. It is most often found at extraocular sites, including the salivary gland, but can be found arising from the conjunctiva and lacrimal system as a distinct mass lesion. The lesions are often rapidly growing and invasive, though they rarely metastasize. Like mucinous eccrine adenocarcinoma, well-differentiated mucoepidermoid carcinomas are known to produce mucin [49].

Other Tumors and Inflammatory Conditions

Sebaceous carcinoma can also mimic other benign sebaceous neoplasms including sebaceous adenomas and sebaceous hyperplasia [26]. Other tumors that may arise in and around the orbit including lymphoma, Merkel cell carcinoma, and metastases should also be considered [2]. Finally, sebaceous carcinoma may also present similarly to inflammatory conditions such sarcoidosis and cicatricial pemphigoid [1].

Histopathology

Histopathological classification of sebaceous carcinoma encompasses four distinct types. These types include lobular sebaceous carcinoma, comedocarcinoma, papillary sebaceous carcinoma, and mixed sebaceous carcinoma, with lobular sebaceous carcinoma being the most common [1, 2, 8, 30]. None of these classifications seem to offer any prognostic differentiation. Instead, more common neoplastic prognostic factors such as size, local invasion, regional and distant metastases seem to correlate with poorer prognosis. Histopathological evaluation can help with staging and evaluation of these prognos-

Fig. 5.3 Full-thickness H&E section showing sebaceous carcinoma with pagetoid invasion of the eyelid epidermis. (Shalin and Lazar [77])

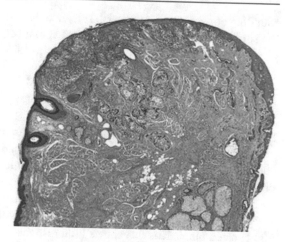

tic factors by assessing for surrounding tissue invasion, including epithelial pagetoid spread and perineural invasion [50]. Tumors with multicentric origins also carry a worse prognosis as they result in a greater risk of local recurrence [2].

Differentiating sebaceous carcinoma from other malignancies can prove difficult without immunohistochemistry staining. An H&E stained section of sebaceous carcinoma of the eyelid is shown in Fig. 5.3. The tumor can often show features of squamous and basal cell carcinoma, which leads to frequent misdiagnosis of sebaceous carcinoma [8]. Common immunohistochemistry stains utilized for detection of sebaceous carcinoma include epithelial membrane antigen [EMA], cytokeratin [Cam 5.2], Ber-EP4, and androgen receptor stain [30]. Staining with adipophilin and perilipin have also shown great promise in aiding in diagnosis of sebaceous carcinoma. Reports have shown adipophilin staining to have a sensitivity and specificity in the detection of sebaceous carcinoma of 97.1% [2].

Sebaceous carcinoma also presents with varied levels of differentiation, from well-differentiated cells to a more poorly differentiated form of the disease. Sebaceous carcinoma can be classified based on cellular differentiation into one of three classes including well-differentiated, moderately differentiated, and poorly differentiated sebaceous carcinoma [1, 2]. Well-differentiated sebaceous cell carcinoma shows histological patterns similar to normal sebaceous glands including vacuolated, frothy cytoplasm with lipid deposits. These cytoplasmic lipid deposits imbue sebaceous carcinoma with its characteristic waxy, yellow color [50]. The organization of sebaceous carcinoma tends to follow a characteristic pattern of differentiated cells located internally, with poorly differentiated cells on the periphery [1]. Poorly differentiated sebaceous carcinoma shows common features of other malignancies including nuclear pleomorphism, increased mitotic activity, and hyperchromatic nuclei [30]. There is a more favorable prognosis for well-differentiated forms of the malignancy compared to the poorly differentiated forms, which are associated with increased mortality rates [29].

Though sebaceous carcinoma may clinically mimic other inflammatory conditions, histopathologically it often shows diminished inflammatory markers compared to other skin cancers including basal and squamous cell carcinomas [1]. In fact, compared to basal cell carcinoma, sebaceous carcinoma has been shown to be free of mononuclear inflammatory cell infiltrates, and seems to show a limited T-cell infiltration of the vasculature surrounding the tumor [51].

The tendency of sebaceous carcinoma to undergo intraepithelial pagetoid spread allows the malignancy to invade surrounding tissues, while making it difficult to localize the invasion [1, 2, 4, 34]. Conjunctival map biopsies are thought to be crucial in determining the extent of spread and, thus, for staging and determining appropriate treatment options. The malignancy is known to invade the surrounding conjunctiva, but can also spread to the corneal epithelium as well. Biopsies must be taken of the surrounding palpebral, forniceal, and bulbar conjunctiva, ideally in a 360-degree fashion, as sebaceous carcinoma is known to spread in a skip-lesion type pattern [50].

Diagnosis

Sebaceous carcinoma's ability to masquerade as different disease processes requires vigilance as a clinician for proper diagnosis. Slit-lamp examination of patients presenting with eyelid complaints should be thorough. Eversion of the eyelids should be performed to evaluate the palpebral and forniceal conjunctiva for evidence of intraepithelial involvement including eyelid thickening and pagetoid spread. Definitive diagnosis of sebaceous carcinoma requires histopathological diagnosis via excisional biopsy [1, 2, 8, 30]. There should be a low threshold for biopsy in cases of recurrent chalazia and chronic blepharitis that shows little response to conventional treatment, especially in the elderly population. Following definitive diagnosis of sebaceous carcinoma, screening should be performed to determine the need for genetic testing to diagnose Muir-Torre syndrome.

Map biopsies are typically performed following definitive diagnosis of periocular sebaceous carcinoma or in cases of suspected tumor recurrence. First described by Putterman in 1986, conjunctival map biopsies can be utilized to determine the presence of intraepithelial pagetoid spread of sebaceous carcinoma [14]. Standard templates for conjunctival map biopsies have been suggested by Putterman and Shields, which sample diffuse areas of the palpebral, bulbar, and forniceal conjunctiva. However, utilizing alternative biopsy sites is important to consider based on the clinical presentation in each patient [52]. Recently, some authors have questioned the usefulness of conjunctival map biopsies, but performing them for sebaceous carcinoma is currently the standard of care for most surgeons [53].

Though regional rates of metastasis of sebaceous carcinoma are around 2.4%, a thorough examination of the cervical, submandibular, parotid, and preaurical lymph nodes should be performed to evaluate for evidence of metastasis. Periocular sebaceous carcinoma seems to metastasize more frequently, at a rate of 4.4% compared to other head and neck sebaceous carcinomas at 0.9%. This difference is likely due in part to the difficulty in diagnosing the periocular form of the disease [54]. Primary metastasis is likely to occur first to the regional lymph nodes, but distant metastases to lung, liver, brain, and bone can occur [55]. Magnetic resonance imaging [MRI] can be utilized to determine the presence and extent of metastasis in patients exhibiting systemic signs of malignancy including weight loss and fatigue. For local invasion, computed tomography [CT] and MRI of the face to examine for invasion of surrounding orbital structures and the sinuses is indicated. If there is evidence of nodal metastasis on exam, a combination of positron emission tomography [PET] scanning and CT scan first be utilized to determine extent of metastasis. Sentinel lymph node biopsy followed by regional lymph node dissection is sometimes performed if evidence of spread on examination is noted [56]. The exact role of sentinel lymph node biopsy is currently debated, though it has been suggested that false negative rates of sentinel lymph node biopsy range from 5% to 25% in periocular tumors, making the value of a negative biopsy inconclusive [57]. There is currently an ongoing clinical trial examining the role of nodal dissection in periocular sebaceous carcinomas to be completed in 2020 [2].

Staging of the disease per the American Joint Committee on Cancer TNM staging guidelines requires data on tumor size, nodal involvement, and distant metastasis. Staging based on these guidelines seems to correlate with disease prognosis. One study found no evidence of nodal metastasis in tumors staged as T2a or smaller than 10 mm in diameter. The authors concluded based on their data that sentinel lymph node biopsies should, thus, be reserved for tumors exceeding these staging criteria [58].

Muir-Torre Syndrome

Muir-Torre syndrome [MTS] is an autosomal dominant genetic condition that predisposes to sebaceous carcinoma, keratoacanthomas, and gastrointestinal malignancies including stomach and duodenal cancers. Roughly half of individuals affected by MTS develop multiple malignancies [11]. Sebaceous carcinomas are extremely common in this group, representing roughly 30% of malignancies, many of which develop in the periocular region [2]. MTS is a variant of Lynch syndrome, or hereditary non-polyposis colorectal cancer [HNPCC], characterized by germ line mutations in DNA mismatch repair [MMR] genes including *MLH1*, *MLH2*, *MSH6*, and *PMS2* [59]. Mutations in these MMR genes lead to an inability to detect base-pairing errors during DNA replication, which result in microsatellite instability of areas of repetitive DNA sequences and an increase in carcinogenesis. Risk factors for development of malignancy in patients with MTS are similar to the risk factors of sebaceous carcinoma including radiation exposure and immunosuppression [60]. These risk factors likely predispose patients to developing a second mutation in the MMR genes in concordance with Knudson's two-hit hypothesis of tumorigenesis [61].

Patients presenting with eyelid sebaceous carcinoma and a positive family history of malignancy including colorectal, genitourinary, and breast cancers should be advised on further genetic testing for diagnosis of MTS. Currently, immunohistochemistry can be utilized to identify sebaceous carcinomas with mutations in the commonly mutated MMR genes, which can be analyzed with reflex immunohistochemistry staining after confirming histopathological diagnosis of sebaceous carcinoma [30]. In line with the Bethesda Guidelines for testing for microsatellite instability in patients suspected of HNPCC [62], Dr. Kyllo and associates created a proposed screening algorithm for patients diagnosed with sebaceous carcinomas. After confirming the diagnosis of sebaceous carcinoma, they suggest the need to gather an in-depth family history of cancer, with a focus on skin and visceral malignancies. Furthermore, given the ease of testing, reflex immunohistochemistry stains should be performed on pathological specimens of confirmed sebaceous carcinoma to identify mutated MMR genes. If either of these screening tools are positive, the patient should be referred to a geneticist for evaluation of microsatellite instability and the presence of possible germ line mutations. A strong primary care relationship should also be established to coordinate frequent cancer screenings including colonoscopies and skin exams. Given the high frequency of multiple malignancies, approaching nearly 40% in patients with MTS, utilization of this screening algorithm has the potential to greatly benefit health outcomes [2].

Recently, an autosomal recessive syndrome that closely resembles MTS has been identified [60]. Coined MUTYHP-associated polyposis (MAP), the syndrome is associated with the development of colorectal adenocarcinomas and sebaceous neoplasms without the characteristic mutations in the MMR genes observed in MTS. Instead, mutations are found in the *MUTYH* gene. This germ line mutation can be missed during analysis of patients for MTS, and must be considered if genetic testing is inconclusive in patients presenting with the phenotypic findings of MTS [63].

Management

Management of sebaceous carcinoma is generally geared towards complete surgical excision of the primary tumor [64, 65]. Given the tendency of sebaceous carcinoma to develop on cosmetically sensitive areas such as the eyelid and face, Mohs micrographic surgery (MMS) has also been successfully employed in treatment of the disease [66]. The choice between utilizing a wide local excision of the primary tumor versus Mohs is a surgeon-specific decision, as evidence is thus far inconclusive regarding rates of recurrence or spread of periocular sebaceous carcinoma between the two approaches [67].

Furthermore, an analysis of several cases in the SEER database showed no difference in overall mortality when comparing the two surgical management techniques [68]. In cases of confirmed intraepithelial pagetoid spread via conjunctival map biopsy, however, MMS is not recommended for management given the diffuse and noncontiguous spread of the malignancy. When choosing wide local excision for primary management on the eyelid, 5–6 mm margins are typically targeted [69]. Other clinicians have suggested utilizing local excision with paraffin histopathological analysis followed by delayed reconstruction to limit the destruction of local tissue, while ensuring adequate removal of involved tissue [50]. In cases of local invasion into the surrounding orbital structures, exenteration is required to prevent further metastasis [1]. As discussed above, SLN biopsy can be performed to determine local metastasis. Confirmed lymph node metastasis requires local lymphadenectomy to help control spread of the malignancy [56, 57].

Topical chemotherapy with mitomycin C has been described for use in sebaceous carcinoma with pagetoid spread. However, the application of topical chemotherapeutic agents to the conjunctiva may result in severe side effects including loss of visual acuity, chronic dry eye, and corneal ulceration [2]. Another option for management of pagetoid spread of sebaceous carcinoma is cryotherapy of the conjunctiva, especially following initial tumor removal and confirmation of spread via map biopsy [1, 8].

Amniotic membrane grafting is another technique employed in reconstruction procedures following surgical excision of ocular tumors involving the conjunctiva [1]. In patients with sebaceous carcinoma characterized by diffuse pagetoid involvement of the conjunctival epithelium, amniotic membrane grafting following broad surgical removal of the involved conjunctiva can help limit the need for more aggressive procedures [70]. Conjunctival autografts and oral mucosal grafts can also be used for conjunctival reconstruction.

For patients whom are not deemed surgical candidates, radiation therapy may be employed. Radiation therapy alone results in increased rates of recurrence compared to surgical excision. Four-year mortality rates in patients undergoing radiation therapy have been reported as high as 78% [30]. However, in one small case report study there were no reports of recurrence in patients receiving greater than 55 Gy of radiation, although it is still advisable for initial management to be centered around surgical excision [2, 71]. In cases of perineural invasion, which carry a diminished prognosis, radiation can be utilized as a postoperative adjuvant therapy [72].

In cases of metastatic sebaceous carcinoma, systemic chemotherapy may be employed to help decrease tumor burden. Distant metastases are rare in sebaceous carcinoma, and there is little evidence for supporting distinct chemotherapy regimens. However, cisplatin-based chemotherapies are most often used in cancers of the head and neck. Some cases have also reported efficacy of 5-flurouracil in managing sebaceous carcinomas [73].

Prognosis

The prognosis for individuals diagnosed with sebaceous carcinoma depends on a variety of factors, especially tumor grade at the time of diagnosis. Other factors identified as individual prognostic indicators include age at time of diagnosis and the presence of distant metastasis [74]. Overall rates of metastasis, including regional nodal and distant metastasis of head and neck sebaceous carcinoma approach nearly 2.5%. However, eyelid carcinomas tend to skew this average higher, as the metastasis rate for this group of cancers is around 4.4% [54]. Rates of distant metastasis of sebaceous carcinoma appear to be less than 1% [74]. Five- and 10-year age-matched survival rates for sebaceous carcinoma are 91.9% and 79.2%, respectively. No statistical difference has been found in survival rates for orbital sebaceous carcinoma versus non-orbital disease [9]. Also, there was no change in rates of disease-specific survival when comparing initial treatment with Mohs micrographic surgery versus wide local excision [74].

Level of differentiation seen on histopathological examination correlates significantly with overall mortality rates. Interestingly, an analysis of the National Cancer Institute's SEER database revealed an increased rate of poorly differentiated eyelid sebaceous carcinoma compared to tumors at other sites of the head and neck region (49.8% vs. 22.7%). Poorly differentiated sebaceous carcinoma was also found to result in increased rates of nodal and distant metastases compared to well-differentiated tumors (13.9% vs. 0%) [54]. However, on multivariate analysis nodal metastasis was noted to not result in a significant increase in cause-specific mortality over and above the increase seen in poorly differentiated sebaceous carcinoma [74].

Other prognostic indicators specific to periocular sebaceous carcinoma include size greater than 10 mm, delayed diagnosis, and upper and lower eyelid involvement [2]. Thus, prompt recognition and diagnosis of this malignancy by ophthalmologists may play a major role in limiting the morbidity and mortality of the disease. The authors recommend frequent follow-up with an ophthalmologist for all patients diagnosed with sebaceous carcinoma, even following surgical removal, especially given the subtle presentation of recurrent sebaceous carcinoma. Evaluation should also include lymph node examination to monitor for signs of nodal metastasis.

Prognosis for patients diagnosed with MTS is likely diminished compared to those with de novo sebaceous carcinomas given the likelihood of developing multiple malignancies. Some reports suggest rates of multiple malignancies as high as 50% in patients with MTS [75]. Thus, those patients diagnosed with MTS should also undergo regular screening for gastrointestinal and skin malignancies via colonoscopy and regular dermatologic examinations.

Conclusion

This chapter has explored the great clinical masquerader, sebaceous carcinoma, including its epidemiology, pathogenesis, origins, clinical presentation, differential diagnosis, histopathology, diagnosis, treatment, and prognosis.

To summarize, sebaceous carcinoma is a malignant neoplasm of the sebaceous glands, which is most often found in the periocular region. Periocular sebaceous carcinoma is frequently found arising from the meibomian glands within the tarsus, especially on the upper eyelid. Other ocular sites include the caruncle, Zeiss glands, eyebrow, and conjunctiva [1, 3, 4, 8]. Risk factors associated with development of sebaceous carcinoma include radiation exposure, HPV infection, and immunosuppression. The pathogenesis of sebaceous carcinoma is still unknown, though HPV infection and the tumor suppressor p53 seem to play a role in its development [20–22]. Some genetic disorders also predispose to the development of sebaceous neoplasms including the autosomal dominant Muir-Torre syndrome. Patients with a family history of sebaceous gastrointestinal neoplasms should be referred for genetic testing to evaluate for this genetic predisposition [2].

The most common presentation of periocular sebaceous carcinoma is a fixed, non-painful eyelid nodule. Still, findings on initial presentation of periocular sebaceous carcinoma can remain subtle given its ability to mimic various common eyelid disorders including chalazia and blepharitis. Other less common inflammatory disorders on the differential should include superior limbic keratoconjunctivitis and sarcoidosis [1, 8, 30]. Findings that should prompt the clinician to consider biopsy include recurrent chalazion, unilateral blepharitis resistant to treatment, madarosis, and diffuse eyelid thickening.

Diagnosis of sebaceous carcinoma requires biopsy and histopathological examination. Immunohistochemistry stains have the ability to assist pathologists in differentiating sebaceous carcinoma from other common eyelid neoplasms, such as basal and squamous cell carcinomas [24]. Other less common neoplasms on the differential include mucinous eccrine gland carcinoma and mucoepidermoid carcinoma [47, 49]. Given the neoplasm's ability to undergo subclinical pagetoid spread, conjunctival map biopsies are recommended to help guide treatment of sebaceous carcinoma [14, 52]. Though metastasis rates remain low, lymph node biopsy and imaging studies can be employed to determine the presence of metastasis [56]. MRI and CT can also help inform surgical approach in cases of locally invasive sebaceous carcinoma.

The mainstay of treatment for sebaceous carcinoma is surgical excision of the primary lesion. Both wide local excision and Mohs micrographic surgery have been successfully employed for surgical management of the ocular neoplasm [64, 68]. Radiation, chemotherapy, and cryotherapy have also been utilized as adjunctive treatment [8, 13]. Overall, prognosis for sebaceous carcinoma is positive with 5-year survival rates around 92% [9]. Still, prompt recognition and diagnosis by the clinician has the ability to greatly affect outcomes in patients presenting with periocular sebaceous carcinoma.

Compliance with Ethical Requirements The authors of this chapter do not have any conflicts of interest to report. The writing of this chapter did not involve any studies with human participants or animals performed by any of the authors.

Bibliography

1. Shields JA, Demirci H, Marr BP, Eagle RC, Shields CL. Sebaceous carcinoma of the ocular region: a review. Surv Ophthalmol. 2005;50(2):103–22.
2. Kyllo RL, Brady KL, Hurst EA. Sebaceous carcinoma: review of the literature. Dermatol Surg. 2015;41(1):1–15.
3. Kass LG, Hornblass A. Sebaceous carcinoma of the ocular adnexa. Surv Ophthalmol. 1989;33(6):477–90.
4. Straatsma BR. Meibomian gland tumors. AMA Arch Ophthalmol. 1956 Jul;56(1):71–93.
5. Ginsberg J. Present status of meibomian gland carcinoma. Arch Ophthalmol Chic Ill 1960. 1965;73:271–7.
6. Galea M, Sharma R, Srinivasan S, Roberts F. Demodex blepharitis mimicking eyelid sebaceous gland carcinoma. Clin Exp Ophthalmol. 2014;42(2):208–10.
7. Kaliki S, Gupta A, Ali MH, Ayyar A, Naik MN. Prognosis of eyelid sebaceous gland carcinoma based on the tumor [T] category of the American Joint Committee on Cancer [AJCC] classification. Int Ophthalmol. 2016;36(5):681–90.
8. Orr CK, Yazdanie F, Shinder R. Current review of sebaceous cell carcinoma. Curr Opin Ophthalmol. 2018;29(5):445–50.
9. Dasgupta T, Wilson LD, Yu JB. A retrospective review of 1349 cases of sebaceous carcinoma. Cancer. 2009;115(1):158–65.
10. Kivelä T, Asko-Seljavaara S, Pihkala U, Hovi L, Heikkonen J. Sebaceous carcinoma of the eyelid associated with retinoblastoma. Ophthalmology. 2001;108(6):1124–8.
11. Dores GM, Curtis RE, Toro JR, Devesa SS, Fraumeni JF. Incidence of cutaneous sebaceous carcinoma and risk of associated neoplasms: insight into Muir-Torre syndrome. Cancer. 2008;113(12):3372–81.
12. Brownstein S, Codere F, Jackson WB. Masquerade syndrome. Ophthalmology. 1980;87(3):259–62.
13. Buitrago W, Joseph AK. Sebaceous carcinoma: the great masquerader: emgerging concepts in diagnosis and treatment. Dermatol Ther. 2008;21(6):459–66.
14. Putterman AM. Conjunctival map biopsy to determine pagetoid spread. Am J Ophthalmol. 1986;102(1):87–90.
15. Khan JA, Doane JF, Grove AS. Sebaceous and meibomian carcinomas of the eyelid. Recognition, diagnosis, and management. Ophthal Plast Reconstr Surg. 1991;7(1):61–6.
16. Lin H-Y, Cheng C-Y, Hsu W-M, Kao WHL, Chou P. Incidence of eyelid cancers in Taiwan: a 21-year review. Ophthalmology. 2006;113(11):2101–7.
17. Lee SB, Saw SM, Au Eong KG, Chan TK, Lee HP. Incidence of eyelid cancers in Singapore from 1968 to 1995. Br J Ophthalmol. 1999;83(5):595–7.
18. Lanoy E, Dores GM, Madeleine MM, Toro JR, Fraumeni JF, Engels EA. Epidemiology of nonkeratinocytic skin cancers among persons with AIDS in the United States. AIDS Lond Engl. 2009;23(3):385–93.
19. Harwood CA, Swale VJ, Bataille VA, Quinn AG, Ghali L, Patel SV, et al. An association between sebaceous carcinoma and microsatellite instability in immunosuppressed organ transplant recipients. J Invest Dermatol. 2001;116(2):246–53.

20. Thomas M, Pim D, Banks L. The role of the E6-p53 interaction in the molecular pathogenesis of HPV. Oncogene. 1999;18(53):7690–700.
21. Stagner AM, Afrogheh AH, Jakobiec FA, Iacob CE, Grossniklaus HE, Deshpande V, et al. p16 expression is not a surrogate marker for high-risk human papillomavirus infection in periocular sebaceous carcinoma. Am J Ophthalmol. 2016;170:168–75.
22. Shalin SC, Sakharpe A, Lyle S, Lev D, Calonje E, Lazar AJ. p53 staining correlates with tumor type and location in sebaceous neoplasms. Am J Dermatopathol. 2012;34(2):129–35; quiz 136–8.
23. Hussain RM, Matthews JL, Dubovy SR, Thompson JM, Wang G. UV-independent p53 mutations in sebaceous carcinoma of the eyelid. Ophthal Plast Reconstr Surg. 2014;30(5):392–5.
24. Jakobiec FA, Mendoza PR. Eyelid sebaceous carcinoma: clinicopathologic and multiparametric immunohisto-chemical analysis that includes adipophilin. Am J Ophthalmol. 2014;157(1):186–208.e2.
25. Hayashi N, Furihata M, Ohtsuki Y, Ueno H. Search for accumulation of p53 protein and detection of human papillomavirus genomes in sebaceous gland carcinoma of the eyelid. Virchows Arch Int J Pathol. 1994;424(5):503–9.
26. Eisen DB, Michael DJ. Sebaceous lesions and their associated syndromes: part I. J Am Acad Dermatol. 2009;61(4):549–60; quiz 561–2.
27. Snow SN, Larson PO, Lucarelli MJ, Lemke BN, Madjar DD. Sebaceous carcinoma of the eyelids treated by mohs micrographic surgery: report of nine cases with review of the literature. Dermatol Surg. 2002;28(7):623–31.
28. Wolfe JT, Yeatts RP, Wick MR, Campbell RJ, Waller RR. Sebaceous carcinoma of the eyelid. Errors in clinical and pathologic diagnosis. Am J Surg Pathol. 1984;8(8):597–606.
29. Rao NA, Hidayat AA, McLean IW, Zimmerman LE. Sebaceous carcinomas of the ocular adnexa: a clinicopathologic study of 104 cases, with five-year follow-up data. Hum Pathol. 1982;13(2):113–22.
30. Knackstedt T, Samie FH. Sebaceous carcinoma: a review of the scientific literature. Curr Treat Options in Oncol. 2017;18(8):47.
31. Mebazaa A, Boussofara L, Trabelsi A, Denguezli M, Sriha B, Belajouza C, et al. Undifferentiated sebaceous carcinoma: an unusual childhood cancer. Pediatr Dermatol. 2007;24(5):501–4.
32. Boniuk M, Zimmerman LE. Sebaceous carcinoma of the eyelid, eyebrow, caruncle, and orbit. Trans Am Acad Ophthalmol Otolaryngol. 1968;72(4):619–42.
33. Pandey K, Singh P, Singh A, Pandey H. Primary sebaceous gland carcinoma of the bulbar conjunctiva without involvement of eyelid: a clinical dilemma. Oman J Ophthalmol. 2011;4(2):97–9.
34. Wick MR, Goellner JR, Wolfe JT, Su WP. Adnexal carcinomas of the skin. II. Extraocular sebaceous carcinomas. Cancer. 1985;56(5):1163–72.
35. Aung PP, Batrani M, Mirzabeigi M, Goldberg LJ. Extraocular sebaceous carcinoma in situ: report of three cases and review of the literature. J Cutan Pathol. 2014;41(7):592–6.
36. Candelario NM, Sánchez JE, Sánchez JL, Martín-García RF, Rochet NM. Extraocular sebaceous carcinoma-a clinicopathologic reassessment. Am J Dermatopathol. 2016;38(11):809–12.
37. Wellens L, Van Ginderdeuren R, Mombaerts I. Chronic blepharitis. Int J Dermatol. 2018;57(12):1437–8.
38. Callahan EF, Appert DL, Roenigk RK, Bartley GB. Sebaceous carcinoma of the eyelid: a review of 14 cases. Dermatol Surg. 2004;30(8):1164–8.
39. Barsegian A, Shinder R. Eyelid sebaceous gland carcinoma with extensive pagetoid spread. Ophthalmology. 2017;124(6):858.
40. Yang PT, Tucker NA, Rootman DB, Rootman DS, McGowan H, Chan CC. Pagetoid spread of sebaceous cell carcinoma to the cornea. Can J Ophthalmol. 2012;47(6):e46–7.
41. Zaragoza P. Intraepithelial sebaceous gland carcinoma with pagetoid spread presenting as marginal keratitis: a case report. Eye Lond Engl. 2003;17(4):536–7.
42. Sainz de la Maza M, Foster CS. Peripheral ulcerative keratitis and malignancies. Cornea. 1994;13(4):364–7.
43. Condon GP, Brownstein S, Codère F. Sebaceous carcinoma of the eyelid masquerading as superior limbic keratoconjunctivitis. Arch Ophthalmol Chic Ill 1960. 1985;103(10):1525–9.
44. Reifler DM, Hornblass A. Squamous cell carcinoma of the eyelid. Surv Ophthalmol. 1986;30(6):349–65.
45. Margo CE, Waltz K. Basal cell carcinoma of the eyelid and periocular skin. Surv Ophthalmol. 1993;38(2):169–92.
46. Shields CL, Kels JG, Shields JA. Melanoma of the eye: revealing hidden secrets, one at a time. Clin Dermatol. 2015;33(2):183–96.
47. Durairaj VD, Hink EM, Kahook MY, Hawes MJ, Paniker PU, Esmaeli B. Mucinous eccrine adenocarcinoma of the periocular region. Ophthal Plast Reconstr Surg. 2006;22(1):30–5.
48. Koch KR, Ortmann M, Heindl LM. Conjunctival Mucoepidermoid Carcinoma. Ophthalmology. 2016;123(3):616.
49. Singh L, Singh S, Jain D, Sharma SC. Mucoepidermoid carcinoma of eyelid: a usual tumor at an unusual site. J Cancer Res Ther. 2015;11(4):1027.
50. While B, Salvi S, Currie Z, Mudhar HS, Tan JHY. Excision and delayed reconstruction with paraffin section histopathological analysis for periocular sebaceous carcinoma. Ophthal Plast Reconstr Surg. 2014;30(2):105–9.

51. Herman DC, Chan CC, Bartley GB, Nussenblatt RB, Palestine AG. Immunohistochemical staining of sebaceous cell carcinoma of the eyelid. Am J Ophthalmol. 1989;107(2):127–32.

52. McConnell LK, Syed NA, Zimmerman MB, Carter KD, Nerad JA, Allen RC, et al. An analysis of conjunctival map biopsies in sebaceous carcinoma. Ophthal Plast Reconstr Surg. 2017;33(1):17–21.

53. Sa H-S, Tetzlaff MT, Esmaeli B. Predictors of local recurrence for eyelid sebaceous carcinoma: questionable value of routine conjunctival map biopsies for detection of pagetoid spread. Ophthal Plast Reconstr Surg. 2019;35(5):419–25.

54. Tryggvason G, Bayon R, Pagedar NA. Epidemiology of sebaceous carcinoma of the head and neck: implications for lymph node management. Head Neck. 2012;34(12):1765–8.

55. Song A, Carter KD, Syed NA, Song J, Nerad JA. Sebaceous cell carcinoma of the ocular adnexa: clinical presentations, histopathology, and outcomes. Ophthal Plast Reconstr Surg. 2008;24(3):194–200.

56. Pfeiffer ML, Savar A, Esmaeli B. Sentinel lymph node biopsy for eyelid and conjunctival tumors: what have we learned in the past decade? Ophthal Plast Reconstr Surg. 2013;29(1):57–62.

57. Ho VH, Ross MI, Prieto VG, Khaleeq A, Kim S, Esmaeli B. Sentinel lymph node biopsy for sebaceous cell carcinoma and melanoma of the ocular adnexa. Arch Otolaryngol Head Neck Surg. 2007;133(8):820–6.

58. Esmaeli B, Nasser QJ, Cruz H, Fellman M, Warneke CL, Ivan D. American Joint Committee on Cancer T category for eyelid sebaceous carcinoma correlates with nodal metastasis and survival. Ophthalmology. 2012;119(5):1078–82.

59. Cornejo KM, Hutchinson L, Deng A, Tomaszewicz K, Welch M, Lyle S, et al. BRAF/KRAS gene sequencing of sebaceous neoplasms after mismatch repair protein analysis. Hum Pathol. 2014;45(6):1213–20.

60. John AM, Schwartz RA. Muir-Torre syndrome [MTS]: an update and approach to diagnosis and management. J Am Acad Dermatol. 2016;74(3):558–66.

61. Berger AH, Knudson AG, Pandolfi PP. A continuum model for tumour suppression. Nature. 2011;476(7359):163–9.

62. Umar A, Boland CR, Terdiman JP, Syngal S, de la Chapelle A, Rüschoff J, et al. Revised Bethesda guidelines for hereditary nonpolyposis colorectal cancer [Lynch syndrome] and microsatellite instability. J Natl Cancer Inst. 2004;96(4):261–8.

63. Kacerovska D, Drlik L, Slezakova L, Michal M, Stehlik J, Sedivcova M, et al. Cutaneous sebaceous lesions in a patient with MUTYH-associated polyposis mimicking Muir-Torre syndrome. Am J Dermatopathol. 2016;38(12):915–23.

64. Cook BE, Bartley GB. Treatment options and future prospects for the management of eyelid malignancies: an evidence-based update. Ophthalmology. 2001;108(11):2088–98; quiz 2099–100, 2121.

65. Shields JA, Saktanasate J, Lally SE, Carrasco JR, Shields CL. Sebaceous carcinoma of the ocular region: the 2014 professor Winifred Mao lecture. Asia Pac J Ophthalmol Phila Pa. 2015;4(4):221–7.

66. Brady KL, Hurst EA. Sebaceous carcinoma treated with Mohs micrographic surgery. Dermatol Surg. 2017;43(2):281–6.

67. Hou JL, Killian JM, Baum CL, Otley CC, Roenigk RK, Arpey CJ, et al. Characteristics of sebaceous carcinoma and early outcomes of treatment using Mohs micrographic surgery versus wide local excision: an update of the Mayo Clinic experience over the past 2 decades. Dermatol Surg. 2014;40(3):241–6.

68. Phan K, Loya A. Mohs micrographic surgery versus wide local excision for sebaceous adenocarcinoma of the eyelid : analysis of a national database. J Plast Reconstr Aesthetic Surg: JPRAS. 2019;72(6):1007–11.

69. Spencer JM, Nossa R, Tse DT, Sequeira M. Sebaceous carcinoma of the eyelid treated with Mohs micrographic surgery. J Am Acad Dermatol. 2001;44(6):1004–9.

70. Tanaka TS, Demirci H. Cryopreserved ultra-thick human amniotic membrane for conjunctival surface reconstruction after excision of conjunctival tumors. Cornea. 2016;35(4):445–50.

71. Yen MT, Tse DT, Wu X, Wolfson AH. Radiation therapy for local control of eyelid sebaceous cell carcinoma: report of two cases and review of the literature. Ophthal Plast Reconstr Surg. 2000;16(3):211–5.

72. Connor M, Droll L, Ivan D, Cutlan J, Weber RS, Frank SJ, et al. Management of perineural invasion in sebaceous carcinoma of the eyelid. Ophthal Plast Reconstr Surg. 2011;27(5):356–9.

73. Kumar V, Xu Y. Unusual presentation of metastatic sebaceous carcinoma and its response to chemotherapy: is genotyping a right answer for guiding chemotherapy in rare tumours? Curr Oncol Tor Ont. 2015;22(4):e316–9.

74. Thomas WW, Fritsch VA, Lentsch EJ. Population-based analysis of prognostic indicators in sebaceous carcinoma of the head and neck. Laryngoscope. 2013;123(9):2165–9.

75. Ponti G, Ponz de Leon M. Muir-Torre syndrome. Lancet Oncol. 2005;6(12):980–7.

76. Schmitz EJ, Herwig-Carl MC, Holz FG, et al. Sebaceous gland carcinoma of the ocular adnexa - variability in clinical and histological appearance with analysis of immunohistochemical staining patterns. Graefes Arch Clin Exp Ophthalmol. 2017;255:2277.

77. Shalin S, Lazar AJF. Sebaceous carcinoma. In: Massi D, editor. Dermatopathology. Encyclopedia of pathology. Cham: Springer; 2016.

Medical Management of Blepharitis

Farida E. Hakim and Asim V. Farooq

Introduction

Broadly, medical management of blepharitis aims to relieve symptoms and to reduce inflammation. There is no established "cure" for blepharitis. The mainstay of treatment for both anterior and posterior blepharitis is daily eyelid hygiene, which includes warm compresses, eyelid massage, gentle eyelid and eyelash scrubs, and artificial tears. Acute exacerbations or severe chronic disease may require treatment with topical steroids, topical antibiotics, topical steroid/antibiotic combination therapy, topical calcineurin inhibitors, or oral antibiotics. It is prudent to adopt a stepwise approach starting with lid hygiene and escalating to oral medications or combination therapy in refractory cases. It is also critical that patients understand the chronic nature of blepharitis and that some degree of daily treatment may be required to control inflammation and symptoms [1, 2].

This chapter discusses the medical management options for blepharitis. While anatomy and pathophysiology provide a framework for categorizing blepharitis, there is considerable overlap in the approaches to treatment.

Eyelid Hygiene

Eyelid hygiene consists of warm compresses, eyelid massage, and gentle eyelid/eyelash scrubs. Warm compresses involve the use of hot water on a clean washcloth, over-the-counter eye mask or heat pack, or homemade mask using uncooked rice or beans. The warm compress is applied one to two times daily to soften adherent lid debris and to warm meibomian gland secretions. Patients should be cautioned against using excessive heat that may burn skin. Eyelid massage is performed with gentle pressure applied to eyelids in a vertical motion against the globe to promote expression of meibomian gland contents. Eyelid and eyelash scrubs remove lid margin debris and substance obstructing meibomian gland orifices, and scurf or scale adherent to lashes [2]. Patients who wear cosmetics around the eyes should be counseled on the importance of removing makeup daily after use. A variety of dedicated eyelid cleansers are available, in the form of gels, foams, sprays, and disposable wipes [3].

F. E. Hakim · A. V. Farooq (✉)
University of Chicago, Chicago, IL, USA
e-mail: afarooq@bsd.uchicago.edu

© Springer Nature Switzerland AG 2021
A. V. Farooq, J. J. Reidy (eds.), *Blepharitis*, Essentials in Ophthalmology,
https://doi.org/10.1007/978-3-030-65040-7_6

There is insufficient evidence to establish one product as superior or more efficacious than another or to establish an ideal regimen for the use of these products [3, 4]. Most are used once or twice a day. In addition to the mechanical disruption and removal of eyelid margin debris and pathogens, cleansers contain ingredients with antimicrobial properties such as hypochlorous acid, tea tree oil, or other active ingredients, which serve to reduce the bacterial or parasitic burden in blepharitis [3]. Dilute baby shampoo has previously been recommended as a convenient, easily obtainable option for performing lid scrubs. However, compared to dedicated eyelid cleansers, the therapeutic effects may be "offset" by the presence of pro-inflammatory agents or irritants to the ocular surface in shampoo. In a randomized double-masked trial comparing TheratearsSteriLid to baby shampoo, levels of MUC5AC expression, a marker of goblet cell density and function in the conjunctival epithelium, were observed to be decreased following 4 weeks of baby shampoo treatment. Increased meibomian gland capping, suggestive of inflammation-induced epithelialization of meibomian gland orifices, was also noted in eyes treated with baby shampoo [5].

Anterior Blepharitis

Staphylococcal Blepharitis

Treatment of staphylococcal blepharitis includes lid hygiene, especially lid scrubs. For acute exacerbations, a topical antibiotic ointment such as erythromycin or bacitracin can be applied to the eyelids one to two times daily for 2–8 weeks, with dosing and duration dependent on severity of presentation and response to treatment. The goal of antibiotic therapy is to reduce inflammation by reducing bacterial load [1, 2, 6].

Topical antibiotic/corticosteroid combinations are also effective therapies for rapidly quelling inflammation, and these medications are available as ointments and ophthalmic suspensions. Dexamethasone 0.1%/tobramycin 0.3% and loteprednol etabonate 0.5%/tobramycin 0.3% administered four times per day for 14 days have been demonstrated to be equally effective in treating blepharoconjunctivitis. Loteprednol etabonate is a less potent corticosteroid than dexamethasone and carries a lower risk of steroid-induced intraocular pressure elevation [1].

Seborrheic Blepharitis

As with staphyloccocal blepharitis, the treatment for seborrheic blepharitis consists of lid hygiene and topical antibiotics and topical steroids if needed.

Demodicosis

Warm compresses, topical antibiotics, and steroids alone are ineffective for treating demodex blepharitis [7, 8]. If blepharitis does not improve with these therapies, *Demodex* should be suspected. While there is no standard treatment in terms of formulation or frequency, existing treatments appear to be effective by reducing parasitic burden [8]. Tea tree oil, an extract from the leaves of the *Melaleuca alternifolia* plant, has been found to be an effective treatment in a variety of formulations including ointments, shampoo, and facewash, providing both symptom relief and decreasing mite count [9–11]. The active acaracidal ingredient, terpinen-4-ol, may provide effective treatment without other irritants in tea tree oil [12, 13]. This compound kills mites but not eggs, so it may be beneficial to do at least 2 rounds of treatment 2 weeks apart, which accounts for the *Demodex* life cycle [11].

In a small study, 5% permethrin cream daily to lids, lashes, and brows was also shown to reduce the number of mites on lashes; however, there was not a significant effect on patient symptoms [14]. Further investigation is needed.

Honey is another natural substance garnering attention for anti-inflammatory and anti-microbial properties, attributed to low pH, high osmolarity, hydrogen peroxide content, and non-peroxide substances including methylglyoxal (MGO). New Zealand native Manuka honey (*Leptospermum scoparium*) has been the subject of interest as a potential anti-inflammatory agent for blepharitis and other skin conditions due to its high MGO content [15]. An augmented Manuka honey formulation demonstrated comparable efficacy to 50% tea tree oil in killing *Demodex* mites in an in vitro study [15]. In a small prospective, investigator-masked, randomized, paired-eye trial, a novel Manuka honey microemulsion eye cream yielded significant improvement in ocular surface symptoms and appearance, tear film stability, and *Demodex* burden [16]. Further investigation for this promising therapeutic option is warranted.

In cases that are refractory to topical medications, systemic therapy may be warranted. Ivermectin is a well-known anti-helminthic and anti-parasitic medication that has been demonstrated to be effective against *Demodex*. It selectively binds glutamate-gated chloride ion channels to interfere with neurotransmission in the peripheral nervous system of the organism [8, 17]. Oral administration of 200 micrograms/kg 7 days apart was successful in reducing the number of mites and improving symptoms in patients with blepharitis not responsive to other treatments [18, 19]. Combination therapy with oral metronidazole was also shown to be effective and superior to ivermectin alone, and may also be considered in refractory cases [20].

Ivermectin should be used with caution in patients with cardiac, renal, and liver disease and patients older than 65 years of age as it has not been studied in these populations. Side effects that have been reported include dizziness, headache, nausea, vomiting, and diarrhea; however, no adverse effects were reported in the context of treatment for *Demodex* [8, 17]. It is not recommended for women who are pregnant or breastfeeding and children weighing less than 15 kg as data regarding safety in these populations is not conclusive [17].

Allergic Blepharitis

In cases of contact blepharitis or allergic blepharitis where inflammation is attributed to cosmetics or ophthalmic or dermatologic topical medication, the offending agent should be discontinued [21, 22]. Preservatives in ophthalmic medications such as benzalkonium chloride and thimerosal are frequent offenders. A table of sources of allergic blepharitis can be found in Chapter 1. When blepharitis is secondary to a medication, physicians should seek an alternative medication, such as a preservative-free option [22]. For allergic blepharitis and blepharoconjunctivitis, systemic (cetirizine, diphenhydramine) or topical antihistamines (olopatadine) may be helpful in relieving itch.

Acute exacerbations can be treated with topical calcineurin inhibitors (e.g., cyclosporine ophthalmic emulsion 0.05%), or low-potency topical corticosteroids (e.g., fluorometholone 0.1% or loteprednol etabonate 0.5% ophthalmic suspensions) [23]. In a retrospective chart review, loteprednol ointment 0.5%, FML 0.1%, and DM/T-0.3–0.1% ointment twice daily for 1 month were commonly prescribed and effective regimens [21]. Loteprednol and fluorometholone are corticosteroids with less ocular penetration and lower potency than dexamethasone and are less likely to cause a spike in intraocular pressure (IOP) [1].

Atopic Blepharitis

In both allergic and atopic blepharitis and periocular dermatitis, controlling itch is essential to healing and breaking the cycle of inflammation, as the mechanical injury from rubbing skin leads to the release of pro-inflammatory cytokines. Cool compresses and adequate moisturizer are non-pharmaceutical but essential foundational measures in providing relief [22]. While topical steroids are extremely effective at relieving inflammation, they can cause elevated IOP, posterior subcapsular cataracts, atrophy of the delicate skin of eyelids, and HSV reactivation. There is burgeoning evidence that topical calcineurin inhibitors, tacrolimus and pimecrolimus, applied daily to eyelids or even to the fornix are efficacious in treating atopic blepharitis and have a favorable safety profile [24–26].

Posterior Blepharitis

Meibomian Gland Dysfunction

The vicious pathophysiologic cycle of events that characterizes meibomian gland dysfunction offers several approaches to try to manage this condition. Abnormally functioning meibomian glands (either due to obstruction or pre-existing inflammation causing hyperkeratinization) leads to stasis and thickening of meibum and bacterial colonization of the glands. Release of lipolytic enzymes by bacteria alters the composition of the meibum resulting in both poor expression and further obstruction of the glands as well the release of irritating free fatty acids, all compromising tear film integrity and stability [1, 27]. The consequent evaporative dry eye syndrome worsens ocular surface inflammation. As with anterior blepharitis, warm compresses, eyelid massage, and lid scrubs are mainstays of treatment and important initial interventions. These maneuvers help remove inflammatory debris and work to open obstructed meibomian glands.

Dietary supplementation of fatty acids has been shown to improve dry eye symptoms [1, 28]. It has been hypothesized that dietary supplementation may be beneficial for MGD by altering meibum composition and modulating the local and systemic inflammatory milieu. In one study, dietary supplementation with omega-3 fatty acids (flaxseed oil) led to improved tear break-up time (TBUT), meibum quality, and Ocular Surface Disease Index (OSDI) scores; however, this topic remains controversial [28]. Further investigation is needed to establish a role for fatty acid supplementation in the management of MGD.

Azithromycin and doxycycline are antibiotics that have been shown to improve symptoms and signs of MGD [27, 29–32]. In addition to antimicrobial properties, both demonstrate anti-inflammatory activity. Azithromycin suppresses the production of pro-inflammatory mediators such as TNFa and IL-1β, and numerous matrix metalloproteinases [27]. Doxycycline decreases the activity of phospholipase A2 and reduces the production of interleukin IL-1α and tumor necrosis factor (TNF)-α in corneal epithelium [30].

Topical azithromycin is available in the USA as a 1% ophthalmic solution (Azasite, Inspire Pharmaceuticals, Inc., Durham, NC, USA), and outside the USA as a 1.5% ophthalmic solution (Azyter, Thea Laboratories, France). Azasite is formulated with a polycarbophil-based excipient that prolongs the time the drug is on the ocular surface. Topical administration may even be superior to oral azithromycin, as a high ocular tissue concentration is achieved, without accumulating systemically [33, 34]. Therapeutic levels persist for several days in the conjunctiva after the last dose. Dosing for topical azithromycin is BID for the first 2–3 days then daily for 4 weeks. Oral azithromycin dosing varies but is given either as a pulse with 500 mg to 1 g PO once a week for 3 weeks or a brief 5-day course of 500 mg the first day and 250 mg/day for 4 days [1, 31, 32]. Doxycycline dosing ranges from 40 to 200 mg/day for 3–8 weeks.

Given the risk of adverse systemic effects, oral antibiotics should be used in cases refractory to topical therapy. Oral azithromycin may rarely cause hepatotoxicity, and more commonly may cause nausea, vomiting, diarrhea, and gastrointestinal discomfort [34]. Like other macrolide antibiotics, it can cause QT interval prolongation and torsades de pointes, which is potentially fatal. This medication should be used with caution in patients prone to cardiac arrhythmia as well as patients taking other medications that cause QT prolongation. Doxycycline is known to cause gastrointestinal irritation, including ulceration and esophagitis. It can cause photosensitivity and patients should be counseled to avoid prolonged sun and UV light exposure and to protect skin with sunscreen or clothing. This medication is also associated with intracranial hypertension and patients with pre-existing intracranial hypertension, or women of childbearing age, or patients who are overweight, are at higher risk of this adverse effect [35].

Rosacea

Rosacea is a multi-factorial inflammatory condition affecting the facial skin, and 20% of patients can have ocular disease before any other cutaneous manifestations [36]. Given the chronic nature of this condition, management incorporates both lifestyle modifications as well as adjunctive medical therapies. Diet, climate, and activity-related factors may all contribute to the disease and patients may be advised to keep a log of possible triggering factors. Additional management includes lid hygiene, oral omega-3 supplementation, topical cyclosporine, topical antibiotics (azithromycin, metronidazole, ivermectin), and oral antibiotics in refractory cases [36, 37].

The efficacy of oral azithromycin and doxycycline is thought to be due to anti-inflammatory and immunomodulatory activity, with studies demonstrating decreases in levels of matrix metalloproteinases, interleukins, and other cytokines in the tear film and ocular surface. In fact, oral doxycycline improved the signs and symptoms of rosacea at a sub-antimicrobial dose of 40 mg daily. This lower dose is well tolerated, with a lower chance of adverse effects, and is the only dose approved for use for 16 weeks [38]. Topical therapies are advantageous as they reduce dependence on systemic medications with possible adverse effects such as with doxycycline. Topical azithromycin (1.5% b.i.d. for 6 days) was found to be comparable to oral doxycycline (100 mg/day for 1 month) for treating ocular rosacea [34]. Cyclosporine is a calcineurin inhibitor and ultimately inhibits T-cell activation and the release of pro-inflammatory cytokines. Topical cyclosporine 0.05% twice a day has been shown to provide significant symptom relief and improvement in signs of ocular rosacea compared to artificial tears and compared to oral doxycycline [39, 40].

As *Demodex* has been implicated in rosacea, treatments for this condition may also be helpful in treating ocular rosacea [7, 37]. While brimonidine is a commonly prescribed as an ophthalmic solution for glaucoma, this formulation has not been showed to have an impact on the blepharitis or telangiectasias seen in rosacea. Rather, topical brimonidine 0.5% is shown to reduce facial erythema in rosacea through alpha-adrenergic agonistic action upon vessels of superficial and deep dermal plexuses [41, 42].

Compliance with Ethical Requirements Farida E. Hakim declares that she has no conflict of interest. Asim V. Farooq is a consultant to GlaxoSmithKline. No human or animal studies were carried out by the authors for this chapter.

References

1. Pflugfelder SC, Karpecki PM, Perez VL. Treatment of blepharitis: recent clinical trials. Ocul Surf. 2014;12(4):273–84.
2. Blepharitis PPP-2018 [Internet]. American Academy of Ophthalmology. 2018 [cited 2020 May 28]. Available from: https://www.aao.org/preferred-practice-pattern/blepharitis-ppp-2018.

3. Bitton E, Ngo W, Dupont P. Eyelid hygiene products: a scoping review. Cont Lens Anterior Eye. 2019;42(6):591–7.
4. Murphy O, O'Dwyer V, Lloyd-McKernan A. The efficacy of tea tree face wash, 1, 2-Octanediol and microblepharoexfoliation in treating Demodex folliculorum blepharitis. Cont Lens Anterior Eye. 2018;41(1):77–82.
5. Sung J, Wang MTM, Lee SH, Cheung IMY, Ismail S, Sherwin T, et al. Randomized double-masked trial of eyelid cleansing treatments for blepharitis. Ocul Surf. 2018;16(1):77–83.
6. Lindsley K, Matsumura S, Hatef E, Akpek EK. Interventions for chronic blepharitis. Cochrane Database Syst Rev [Internet]. 2012 [cited 2020 May 27];2012(5). Available from: https://www.ncbi.nlm.nih.gov/pmc/articles/PMC4270370/.
7. Fromstein SR, Harthan JS, Patel J, Opitz DL. Demodex blepharitis: clinical perspectives. Clin Optom (Auckl). 2018;10:57–63.
8. Navel V, Mulliez A, Benoist d'Azy C, Baker JS, Malecaze J, Chiambaretta F, et al. Efficacy of treatments for Demodex blepharitis: a systematic review and meta-analysis. Ocul Surf. 2019;17(4):655–69.
9. Gao Y-Y, Xu D, Huang l-J, Wang R, Tseng SCG. Treatment of ocular itching associated with ocular demodicosis by 5% tea tree oil ointment. Cornea. 2012;31(1):14–7.
10. Karakurt Y, Zeytun E. Evaluation of the efficacy of tea tree oil on the density of Demodex mites (Acari: Demodicidae) and ocular symptoms in patients with demodectic blepharitis. J Parasitol. 2018;104(5):473–8.
11. Evren Kemer Ö, Esra Karaca E, Özek D. Efficacy of cyclic therapy with terpinen-4-ol in Demodex blepharitis: is treatment possible by considering Demodex's life cycle? Eur J Ophthalmol. 2020:1120672120919085.
12. Tighe S, Gao Y-Y, Tseng SCG. Terpinen-4-ol is the most active ingredient of tea tree oil to kill Demodex mites. Transl Vis Sci Technol. 2013;2(7):2.
13. Messaoud R, El Fekih L, Mahmoud A, Ben Amor H, Bannour R, Doan S, et al. Improvement in ocular symptoms and signs in patients with Demodex anterior blepharitis using a novel terpinen-4-ol (2.5%) and hyaluronic acid (0.2%) cleansing wipe. Clin Ophthalmol. 2019;13:1043–54.
14. Hecht I, Melzer-Golik A, Sadi Szyper N, Kaiserman I. Permethrin cream for the treatment of Demodex blepharitis. Cornea. 2019;38(12):1513–8.
15. Frame K, Cheung IMY, Wang MTM, Turnbull PR, Watters GA, Craig JP. Comparing the in vitro effects of MGO™ Manuka honey and tea tree oil on ocular Demodex viability. Cont Lens Anterior Eye. 2018;41(6):527–30.
16. Craig JP, Cruzat A, Cheung IMY, Watters GA, Wang MTM. Randomized masked trial of the clinical efficacy of MGO Manuka Honey microemulsion eye cream for the treatment of blepharitis. Ocul Surf. 2020;18(1):170–7.
17. Ashour DS. Ivermectin: from theory to clinical application. Int J Antimicrob Agents. 2019;54(2):134–42.
18. Holzchuh FG, Hida RY, Moscovici BK, Villa Albers MB, Santo RM, Kara-José N, et al. Clinical treatment of ocular Demodex folliculorum by systemic ivermectin. Am J Ophthalmol. 2011;151(6):1030–1034.e1.
19. Filho PAN, Hazarbassanov RM, Grisolia ABD, Pazos HB, Kaiserman I, Gomes JÁP. The efficacy of oral ivermectin for the treatment of chronic blepharitis in patients tested positive for Demodex spp. Br J Ophthalmol. 2011;95(6):893–5.
20. Salem DA-B, El-Shazly A, Nabih N, El-Bayoumy Y, Saleh S. Evaluation of the efficacy of oral ivermectin in comparison with ivermectin-metronidazole combined therapy in the treatment of ocular and skin lesions of Demodex folliculorum. Int J Infect Dis. 2013;17(5):e343–7.
21. Chisholm SAM, Couch SM, Custer PL. Etiology and management of allergic eyelid dermatitis. Ophthalmic Plast Reconstr Surg. 2017;33(4):248–50.
22. Wolf R, Orion E, Tüzün Y. Periorbital (eyelid) dermatides. Clin Dermatol. 2014;32(1):131–40.
23. Hsu JI, Pflugfelder SC, Kim SJ. Ocular complications of atopic dermatitis. Cutis. 2019;104(3):189–93.
24. Remitz A, Virtanen HM, Reitamo S, Kari O. Tacrolimus ointment in atopic blepharoconjunctivitis does not seem to elevate intraocular pressure. Acta Ophthalmol. 2011;89(3):e295–6.
25. Sakarya Y, Sakarya R. Treatment of refractory atopic blepharoconjunctivitis with topical tacrolimus 0.03% dermatologic ointment. J Ocul Pharmacol Ther. 2012;28(1):94–6.
26. Kiiski V, Remitz A, Reitamo S, Mandelin J, Kari O. Long-term safety of topical pimecrolimus and topical tacrolimus in atopic blepharoconjunctivitis. JAMA Dermatol. 2014;150(5):571–4.
27. Opitz DL, Tyler KF. Efficacy of azithromycin 1% ophthalmic solution for treatment of ocular surface disease from posterior blepharitis. Clin Exp Optom. 2011;94(2):200–6.
28. Macsai MS. The role of omega-3 dietary supplementation in blepharitis and meibomian gland dysfunction (an AOS thesis). Trans Am Ophthalmol Soc. 2008;106:336–56.
29. Foulks GN, Borchman D, Yappert M, Kakar S. Topical azithromycin and oral doxycycline therapy of meibomian gland dysfunction: a comparative clinical and spectroscopic pilot study. Cornea. 2013;32(1):44–53.
30. Zandian M, Rahimian N, Soheilifar S. Comparison of therapeutic effects of topical azithromycin solution and systemic doxycycline on posterior blepharitis. Int J Ophthalmol. 2016;9(7):1016–9.
31. Greene JB, Jeng BH, Fintelmann RE, Margolis TP. Oral azithromycin for the treatment of meibomitis. JAMA Ophthalmol. 2014;132(1):121–2.

32. Kashkouli MB, Fazel AJ, Kiavash V, Nojomi M, Ghiasian L. Oral azithromycin versus doxycycline in meibomian gland dysfunction: a randomised double-masked open-label clinical trial. Br J Ophthalmol. 2015;99(2):199–204.
33. Yildiz E, Yenerel NM, Turan-Yardimci A, Erkan M, Gunes P. Comparison of the clinical efficacy of topical and systemic azithromycin treatment for posterior blepharitis. J Ocul Pharmacol Ther. 2018;34(4):365–72.
34. Kagkelaris KA, Makri OE, Georgakopoulos CD, Panayiotakopoulos GD. An eye for azithromycin: review of the literature. Ther Adv Ophthalmol. 2018;10:2515841418783622.
35. Azithromycin and clarithromycin – UpToDate [Internet]. [cited 2020 May 30]. Available from: https://www.upto-date.com/contents/azithromycin-and-clarithromycin?search=azithromycin&source=search_result&selectedTitle=2~145&usage_type=default&display_rank=1#H19.
36. Doxycycline: Drug information – UpToDate [Internet]. [cited 2020 May 30]. Available from: https://www.uptodate.com/contents/doxycycline-drug-information?search=doxy&source=panel_search_result&selectedTitle=1~148&usage_type=panel&kp_tab=drug_general&display_rank=1#F163310.
37. Thiboutot D, Anderson R, Cook-Bolden F, Draelos Z, Gallo RL, Granstein RD, et al. Standard management options for rosacea: the 2019 update by the National Rosacea Society Expert Committee. J Am Acad Dermatol. 2020;82(6):1501–10.
38. Wladis EJ, Adam AP. Treatment of ocular rosacea. Surv Ophthalmol. 2018;63(3):340–6.
39. Sobolewska B, Doycheva D, Deuter C, Pfeffer I, Schaller M, Zierhut M. Treatment of ocular rosacea with once-daily low-dose doxycycline. Cornea. 2014;33(3):257–60.
40. Schechter BA, Katz RS, Friedman LS. Efficacy of topical cyclosporine for the treatment of ocular rosacea. Adv Ther. 2009;26(6):651–9.
41. Arman A, Demirseren DD, Takmaz T. Treatment of ocular rosacea: comparative study of topical cyclosporine and oral doxycycline. Int J Ophthalmol. 2015;8(3):544–9.
42. Two AM, Wu W, Gallo RL, Hata TR. Rosacea: part II. Topical and systemic therapies in the treatment of rosacea. J Am Acad Dermatol. 2015;72(5):761–70.

Procedural Management

Megan Silas, Johnathan Jeffers, and Hassan Shah

Procedures to Treat Blepharitis

Intraductal Probing of Meibomian Glands

For patients who suffer from obstructive meibomian gland dysfunction resulting in lid tenderness, lid margin congestion and evaporative dry eye, intraductal meibomian gland probing (MGP) may be an option. It is felt that this technique helps to relieve intraductal obstruction, allowing for reduced intraductal pressure, improved flow of meibum, and decreased eyelid margin inflammation. This technique was first described in 2010 by Maskin and is explained below [1].

When preforming MGP, topical viscous anesthetic is applied in the inferior conjunctival fornix and eyelid margin. In patients with significant tenderness, 4% lidocaine can also be applied with a cotton-topped applicator to the area to be probed. After appropriate anesthesia is achieved, a bandage contact lens is placed and the patient is brought into the slit lamp. A 1-mm sterile stainless-steel probe (Rhein Medical, Tampa, FL) is held perpendicular to the eyelid margin and passed into the meibomian gland opening and collinear through to meibomian gland. A 2-mm and a 4-mm probe can be used for deeper meibomian gland penetration. At times, a popping or gritty sensation may be felt by the operator which can indicate penetration through an area of intraductal resistance or obstruction from contraction of periductal fibrosis [2]. This has been termed fixed, firm, focal, unyielding resistance (FFFUR) and can be found in both expressible and non-expressible meibomian glands [3]. Mild dot hemorrhage from the ductal orifice is common post-probing and is nearly always self-resolving [1]. After MGP, comorbid conditions, such as aqueous tear deficiency, should be treated as they can precipitate meibomian gland re-occlusion and decrease the duration of treatment effect [2].

Since its initial description, many variations have been proposed to this technique. Wladis recommended obtaining anesthesia through subcutaneous injection with 2% lidocaine with epinephrine and used a hyfrecator tip (Ellman, Oceanside, NY) for probing [4]. Syed et al. performed MGP

M. Silas · H. Shah (✉)
University of Chicago Medical Center, Department of Ophthalmology and Visual Science, Chicago, IL, USA
e-mail: hshah1@bsd.uchicago.edu

J. Jeffers
University of Chicago Pritzker School of Medicine, Chicago, IL, USA

© Springer Nature Switzerland AG 2021
A. V. Farooq, J. J. Reidy (eds.), *Blepharitis*, Essentials in Ophthalmology,
https://doi.org/10.1007/978-3-030-65040-7_7

on a supine patient under an operating microscope, obtaining anesthesia using a combination of 4% lidocaine-soaked cotton pledget and palpebral sub-conjunctival injection. A von Graefe fixation forceps is used for eyelid stabilization [5]. The ultimate goal, however, remains the same: relief of intraductal obstruction, improved flow of meibum, and subsequent decreased eyelid margin inflammation.

Various studies have shown quantitative improvement in meibum lipid levels, [6] meibum viscosity, [6] and tear break up time [7, 8] after MGP in patients who were previously refractory to medical management. Patients also have reported subjective improvement, as measured using the Ocular Surface Disease Index (OSDI) score, at least 3–6 months following treatment [4, 7]. Clinical examinations of patients during routine follow-up after MGP can show decreased eyelid margin vascularization and conjunctival hyperemia [7].

This procedure can be repeated if symptoms recur. However, in the initial study by Maskin, the majority of patients did not require retreatment over a mean follow-up of 11-months. At this time, long-term efficacy data is limited. Maskin et al. suggested using MGP as a preliminary treatment for MGD as alternative treatments, such as warmth and lid massage, may potentially worsen inflammation by increasing intraductal pressure in the meibomian glands [2].

Vectored Thermal Pulsation

LipiFlow

Vectored thermal pulsation via the LipiFlow device (TearScience, Morrisville, North Carolina, USA) is a recent technology that uses heat and meibomian gland expression. Conventional warm compresses apply heat to the external surface of the eyelid, whereas the LipiFlow System applies direct heat to the upper and lower palpebral eyelids to maximize the heat transfer to the meibomian glands. Simultaneous pulsatile pressure is applied to cutaneous eyelid surfaces to promote expression of melted meibum [9].

Use of the LipiFlow System requires a control system and the single-use activator eyepiece (Fig. 7.1). The eyepiece consists of an eyelid warmer and an eyecup. After application of topical ophthalmic anesthetic, the warmer is placed under the upper and lower eyelids to provide direct heat to the palpebral conjunctiva, reaching temperatures between 41 °C and 43 °C. The eyelids are closed over the eyelid warmer such that the eyecup rests on the anterior cutaneous surface of the eyelids. The eyecup inflates during the treatment session in order to facilitate meibum expression through eyelid massage [9, 10]. Each treatment session lasts 12-minutes and immediately post-treatment patients may notice ocular surface irritation and small subcutaneous eyelid margin hemorrhages [10].

Lane et al. found that a one-time 12-minute treatment with LipiFlow resulted in a statistically significant improvement in meibomian gland secretion and tear break-up time when compared to the conventional warm compress control group. Additionally, patients treated with LipiFlow experienced a greater improvement in dry eye symptoms as determined by decrease in SPEED (Standard Patient Evaluation for Eye Dryness) and OSDI (Ocular Surface Disease Index [11]) scores [9]. However, in this initial study, patients with inflammation or infection were excluded, and thus, LipiFlow may not be ideal for certain types of blepharitis. Patients in this study had sustained improvement for 4 weeks, however there was no long-term follow up regarding the total duration of treatment effect.

Other studies have showed an improvement in symptoms up to 9 months and 1 year following a single treatment [12, 13]. In a prospective, randomized, parallel-group, single-masked study, Hagen et al. showed that a single 12-minute bilateral LipiFlow treatment was superior to a 3-month course of doxycycline at decreasing dry eye symptoms, as measured by SPEED score. Additionally, one session of LipiFlow was at least as effective as daily doxycycline at improving MGD as measured by MG function, TBUT, corneal staining, and conjunctival staining [14].

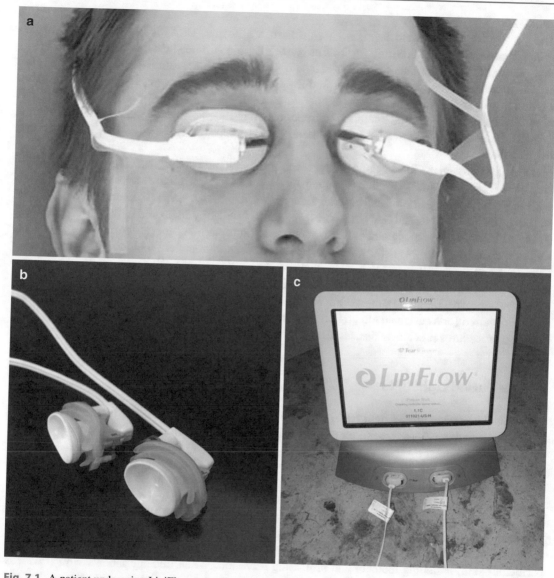

Fig. 7.1 A patient undergoing LipiFlow treatment (**a**). Single-use LipiFlow eyepiece consisting of an eyelid warmer and an eyecup (**b**) and the control system (**c**). (Image courtesy of Blake Williams, MD)

MiBoThermoflo

MiBoThermoflo (MiBo Medical Group, Dallas, Texas, USA) is another in-office device that follows the principle of vectored thermal pulsation by providing external warmth and eyelid massage to facilitate meibum secretion in patients with MGD. Based upon the manufacturer's recommendations, ultrasound gel is applied to the cutaneous surface of the upper and lower eyelid followed by 8–12 minutes of eyelid massage using the handheld probe, which reaches a temperature of 108 °F. The manufacturer recommends that this is repeated every 2 weeks for a total of three sessions. This treatment is operator dependent and relies on the operator ensuring the eyepads are in contact with the anterior eyelids throughout treatment [10]. There has been little data published on the clinical outcomes of patients who have undergone this procedure, however, Kenrick et al. found that the palpebral conjunctival temperature did not reach 40 °C, the required temperature to liquify meibum [15]. Thus, additional research is required to determine the clinical utility of this device.

TearCare

The TearCare System (Sight Sciences, Menlo Park, California, USA) is a recently available in-office treatment for MGD. Similar to LipiFlow, TearCare combines heat and manual eyelid massage to facilitate meibomian gland expression. To administer this treatment, a flexible, single-use iLid is placed externally over the upper and lower tarsal plates of both eyes. Heat is applied for 12 minutes to maintain a therapeutic temperature of 41–45 °C, during which the patient blinks normally to promote natural meibum expression. After the thermal treatment, the meibomian glands are manually expressed using meibomian gland forceps (Rhein Medical Inc., St Petersburg, FL, USA).

The pilot study on the efficacy of this device was a manufacturer sponsored, single-center, randomized trial. The initial study enrolled 24 patients who were randomized to receive a single treatment with the TearCare or daily 5-minute warm compresses. After 4 weeks, TBUT, corneal/conjunctival staining, SPEED, OSDI, and SANDE scores were all significantly improved in the TearCare group. These differences were maintained over 6 months of follow-up and there were no adverse events reported [16]. In a follow-up study, patients received a second treatment 6 months after their initial treatment and were followed for 6 additional months. TBUT improved after retreatment and this effect was sustained for at least 6 months following retreatment [17]. TearCare may be an effective means to improve TBUT and subjective symptoms from MGD, but retreatment at a 6 months interval may be required for a sustained effect. Further studies are necessary to compare TearCare to the other in-office procedures previously discussed.

Intense Pulsed Light (IPL)

Traditionally, intense pulsed light (IPL) has been used for treating vascular or pigmented dermatologic lesions and is FDA-approved for treating telangiectasias [18]. However, it is also used off-label in patients with ocular rosacea and MGD [18].

Initially described by Toyos et al., protective eye pads are placed over closed eyelids, then the entire face is covered in ultrasound gel and is treated with two passes of IPL. After the pulsed light treatment, the meibomian glands are expressed using digital pressure and a cotton-tipped applicator [19]. During IPL treatments, the 500 nm light is absorbed by red blood cells within abnormal telangiectasias resulting in coagulation and thrombosis, preventing the continued secretion of inflammatory mediators from these abnormal vessels. It is also speculated that the heat from the IPL transfers to the periocular skin, softening meibum and promoting secretion. When treating patients with IPL, it is imperative that they be fair skinned (Fitzpatrick Skin Types 1–4), as patients with darker skin are prone to depigmentation. IPL treatment intensity can range from low power (8 J/cm^2) to high power (20 J/cm^2). The physician should start at a lower setting and slowly titrate up based upon disease severity and age [19]. Limitations to this treatment method include cost, as these repeated treatments are is unlikely to be covered by insurance, and patient selection, as only fair-skinned patients are eligible for treatment [18].

A prospective, double-masked, pair-eyed, placebo-controlled study by Craig et al. treated one eye in the inferior periocular area and found statistically significant improvement in symptoms, lipid layer grade, and tear break up time in the treated eye [20]. Additionally, Liu et al. showed decreased levels of IL-17A, IL-6 and PGE2 in eyes treated with IPL when compared to the contralateral control eye indicating that IPL plus meibomian gland expression was more effective than meibomian gland expression alone in reducing inflammation in patients with dry eye disease (DED) and MGD [21]. Thus, although initially described as a potential treatment of MGD, additional studies have found benefits for patients with DED and MGD.

Microblepharoexfoliation

In contrast to many of the abovementioned in-office procedures to treat MGD, the BlephEx device (Scope Ophthalmics, London, UK) is used to target anterior blepharitis as a supplement to home eyelid scrubs. After topical anesthesia is achieved, the BlephEx handpiece is used to spin a single-use, medical grade, micro-sponge while brushing along the eyelash line for 6–8 minutes to remove scurf and debris. After treatment, patients should continue with their home eyelid hygiene regimen. The procedure can be repeated every 4–6 months if symptoms recur. Current studies are limited by small sample size and short-term follow-up; however, preliminary data have shown improvement in TBUT, OSDI scores, MGD and blepharitis, as measured by the Efron Grading Scale [22]. There is also a reduction in matrix metalloproteinase-9 (MMP-9) 4 weeks after treatment with BlephEx [23]. Murphy et al. have shown the BlephEx to be comparable and not statistically superior to OcuSoft Lid Scrub Plus and to Dr. Organic Tea Tree Face Wash in a small randomized study [24].

Surgical Treatment for the Complications of Blepharitis

Chalazia

Chalazia are a common complication of anterior or posterior blepharitis resulting from lipogranulomatous inflammation of obstructed meibomian glands, or the glands of Zeiss and Moll. Initial treatment is conservative, using warm compresses, digital massage, eyelid hygiene, and a combination topical antibiotic-steroid, for inflammation. However, in refractory cases, there are some procedural treatment options.

Steroid Injection

Intralesional steroid injection has been used as a treatment for chalazia for many years [25–28] and has a reported success rates in up to 80% of cases after a single injection [26]. Injections can be administered via a transconjunctival or a transcutaneous approach. Recent reports favor the use of triamcinolone acetonide [26] as the steroid of choice, although methylprednisolone [29] has also been used. The volume, concentration, and injection dose are provider dependent and can vary from 0.02 to 1.0 mL, 5 to 40 mg/mL, and 0.2 to 0.5 mg, respectively [30]. Complications of intralesional steroid injection include periorbital fat atrophy [31], elevated intraocular pressure, tissue hypopigmentation [31], inadvertent globe perforation [32, 33], and infarction of the retinal and choroidal vasculature [29] with or without anterior segment ischemia [34]. Lesion resolution has been reported to occur between 5 days to 3 weeks post injection [30]. Steroid injection can be used alone or in addition to incision and curettage (I&C). When administering after I&C, the chalazion clamp should be left in place for the duration of injection to optimize drug delivery to the affected tissues and decrease the risk of arterial embolization [35].

5-FU Injection

There is an ongoing Phase 3 randomized control trial comparing injection of 5-fluoruracil with steroid injection or I&C for chalazia. This study is actively enrolling, and there are no preliminary data available.

Incision and Curettage (I&C)

I&C is a commonly performed treatment of chalazia refractory to conservative treatments. While surgeon-specific variables exist, the general principle of this treatment is to facilitate drainage of the accumulated lipogranulomatous material. This procedure can be done in an office minor procedure room, or in the operating room if patient cooperation is a concern. It begins with use of topical and infiltrated anesthetic with or without eyelid cleansing with topical 5% betadine. In a transconjunctival approach, the eyelid is clamped and everted for optimal exposure. A vertical incision is made through the conjunctiva to access the accumulated material. If the lesion is more easily accessible via a trans-cutaneous approach, the eyelid is clamped to assist with hemostasis and a horizontal incision is made through the skin over the lesion. The expressed material is cleaned out using cotton-tipped applicators and a chalazion curette. Application of thermal cautery can be used to establish adequate hemostasis. The incision is left open to allow for any residual material to drain. Steroid or antibiotic ointment with or without patching may be used post procedure. The recovery time is minimal and patients can often return to daily activities upon leaving the office.

I&C is the preferred treatment modality for recurrent chalazia because it also allows for biopsy of recurrent chalazia to rule out a malignant lesion such as sebaceous cell carcinoma. This may also be preferred to injection in larger chalazia where the injected medication may not adequately penetrate all tissues involved. Complications of I&C include scarring after transcutaneous incision, inadvertent globe penetration during anesthetic injection, [32] and damage to the puncta or canalicular system in nasal lesions. Additionally, patients may have more apprehension towards an incisional procedure when compared to an eyelid injection.

A large meta-analysis of randomized control trials comparing intralesional steroid with I&C found I&C to be significantly more effective when analyzing resolution after one procedure [30]. I&C was also superior to steroid injection for patients requiring 1 or 2 procedures, but the difference was less substantial. Based upon these results, it appears that a single I&C has a similar success rate as a series of two steroid injections. Individual prospective, randomized studies have shown comparable results between these two modalities [36].

Trichiasis

Trichiasis is a disorder of the eyelid margin where the eyelashes are misdirected towards the globe (Fig. 7.2). There are various etiologies for this acquired disorder, most of which involve chronic inflammation and scarring of the involved eyelash follicle. Blepharitis, through its chronic inflammation of the eyelid margin, has been implicated as well as other inflammatory diseases of the eyelid skin (eczema, atopic disease) or conjunctiva (SJS, OCP, vernal keratoconjunctivitis). First and foremost, treatment should be focused on the etiology of inflammation that is leading to lash misdirection. Once the inflammation is controlled, non-surgical treatments, such as lubrication, bandage contact lens use, or mechanical epilation, may be attempted but are temporary measures. When determining the appro-

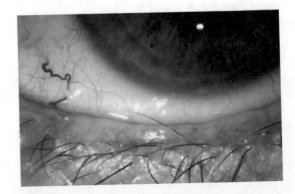

Fig. 7.2 A single misdirected lash in a patient with trichiasis. (From Claudia Auw-Haedrich, Thomas Reinhard. 2008. Chronic Blepharitis: Diagnosis, Pathogenesis, and New Treatment Options. Used with permission of Springer)

priate surgical treatment for trichiasis, it is important to differentiate isolated true trichiasis and trichiasis associated with entropion. For true trichiasis not associated with eyelid malposition, eyelash ablation is preferred.

Radiofrequency Ablation

Radiofrequency ablation is a treatment option for focal or diffuse trichiasis as each lash is treated individually. It employs radiofrequency waves to selectively destroy the adjacent eyelash follicle. This technique was first described by Kezirian in 1993 [37]. After anesthetic infiltration of the affected eyelid, an electrolysis tip is inserted adjacent to the eyelash to the bulb and current is applied for 1–2 seconds. This is repeated until frothing is noted at the eyelid margin. The eyelash can then be easily removed. This procedure is repeated on all affected eyelashes. Post operatively patients are to use antibiotic ointment for 1 week [38].

Electrolysis

Electrolysis is performed using a similar technique as radiofrequency ablation. The affected area is anesthetized with injection of lidocaine with epinephrine. Under the operating microscope, the eyelid is reflected away from the globe, and the electrolysis needle is inserted 2-3 mm deep within the eyelash follicle. Electric current is applied for 1–3 seconds and a whitening of the surrounding skin can be observed. After treatment, the eyelash is then easily removed with forceps. Antibiotic-steroid ointment is recommended post operatively [38, 39]. Sakarya et al. report success with a 55-μm thick ultrafine electrolysis needle. Complications of this procedure include a high rate of recurrence, mild eyelid notching, and faint hypopigmentation [38, 39].

Cryotherapy

Cryotherapy was first reported as a treatment of trichiasis in 1976 and is best used for diffuse trichiasis [40]. This is effective because the hair follicles are more sensitive to the effects of freezing than the skin and conjunctiva [38]. A corneoscleral shell is placed to protect the globe and the eyelid is anesthetized using lidocaine with epinephrine. If a thermocouple is used, it should be inserted through the anterior eyelid skin and orbicularis to reach the pretarsal region just superior to the affected eyelashes. The eyelid margin is moistened with artificial tear gel, and the cryotherapy probe is applied to the eyelashes or to the adjacent palpebral conjunctiva, 2 mm from the eyelid margin, for 20–30 seconds to allow for the tissues to reach −20 to −30 °C as read by the thermocouple. Once the tissues thaw, this is repeated to achieve a double freeze-thaw cycle [38]. Significant eyelid edema and chemosis can be seen in the post-operative period but usually resolves within 5–7 days [41]. Reported complications of cryotherapy include recurrence, madarosis, eyelid notching, palpebral necrosis, skin depigmentation, dry eye syndrome, symblepharon, entropion, and infection [38]. Cryotherapy may be less effective in patients with trichiasis secondary to trachoma due to the extensive conjunctival and tarsal scarring [41].

Laser

Use of various lasers have been reported for the treatment of trichiasis. This is best utilized for eyelids with few misdirected lashes or lashes that are intermittently distributed throughout the eyelid. Argon laser was first used to treat trichiasis in 1979 [42]. This can be performed with topical or infiltrative anesthesia. After appropriate anesthesia is achieved, a corneoscleral shell is placed to protect the globe and the eyelid is everted such that the eyelash follicle is coaxial with the laser beam. Laser settings can vary, but it is suggested to use a 50–200 um spot size and power of 0.2 to 1.5 W for a duration of 200 msec. Multiple shots are applied progressively deeper into the eyelid until the eyelash follicle is destroyed [38, 43]. This procedure is most effective for pigmented eyelashes; however, for nonpigmented eyelashes, black mascara may be applied prior to the procedure to increase effectiveness.

Both the ruby laser (694 nm) [44] and the diode laser (810 nm) [45] have also been described in treating trichiasis, but evidence is limited to small case series. At this time, larger, randomized, comparative studies are needed to determine the efficacy of the various laser options.

Eyelash Trephination

Microtrephination can be used to physically remove the abnormal eyelash follicle. This is best used for small areas of trichiasis with few abnormal lashes. After anesthesia is achieved, a 21-gauge (0.81 mm) Sisler Ophthalmic Microtrephine (Visitec, Sarasota, FL, USA) is placed around the misdirected lash, penetrating 2 mm into the eyelid margin. The abnormal follicle is removed with minimal disruption to the adjacent normal tissue [46]. McCracken et al. felt that this technique induces less inflammation than electrocautery or cryotherapy.

Lamellar Split

Lamellar split is an incisional technique to treat broad areas of trichiasis. The affected eyelid is anesthetized using lidocaine with epinephrine and an incision is made along the gray line to separate the anterior and posterior lamella of the affected area. The anterior and posterior lamellae are dissected apart using a Wescott scissors. The affected lashes can be completely excised and the exposed region closed with a tissue advancement flap [47] or allowed to granulate [48]. Alternatively, monopolar cautery needle can be placed between the anterior and posterior lamellae to cauterize the eyelash follicles. The affected lashes are then removed easily with forceps. The anterior and posterior lamellae are then left to heal by secondary intention [49]. If desired, the lashes be recessed away from the ocular surface as an alternative to complete removal. A free mucous membrane graft is often used with this technique. After dissecting apart the anterior and posterior lamellae, the mucocutaneous graft harvested from the margin of the lip can be placed between the anterior and posterior lamellae to help keep the lashes recessed away from the ocular surface [47].

Wedge Resection

Wedge resection can be used to treat a local area of trichiasis that affects less than 1/3 of the eyelid margin. This can be done in the operating room under light sedation or in a minor procedure room under local anesthesia. The eyelid tissue is infiltrated with lidocaine with epinephrine, and a pentagon-shaped region of the eyelid is removed. If the remaining eyelid is under significant horizontal tension, a lateral cantholysis can be performed to allow for easier approximation [38]. Complications such as pain, bleeding, infection, scar formation, or recurrence can occur with any of the incisional surgeries described.

Distichiasis

Distichiasis is most often a congenital condition where the eyelashes arise from an additional row of cilia posterior to the meibomian glands. However, in patients with chronic inflammation, aberrant lashes may arise from the meibomian gland orifice. The treatment options for distichiasis are similar to that discussed above for trichiasis. However, distichiasis is a much more difficult entity to treat as the aberrant lashes arise from the posterior lamella, and so cannot be separated from the tarsus. There are various advanced surgical procedures described for treatment of distichiasis specifically, but these are beyond the scope of this discussion.

Evaporative Dry Eye

Many patients with meibomian gland dysfunction suffer from evaporative dry eye disease [50, 51]. These patients may benefit from punctal occlusion or closure, especially in the setting of concomitant aqueous deficiency. The concept of punctal plugs was initially described in 1975 with the intention of increased tear retention for aqueous deficiency dry eye [52]. In patients with evaporative dry eye and active inflammation, the traditional teaching has been to avoid punctal plugs or to treat the inflammation prior to placement of punctal plugs to prevent retention of inflammatory cytokines [52]. A recent study by Tong et al. evaluated the levels of 15 cytokines and matrix metalloproteinase-9 in the tear film of patients after placement of punctal plugs and found no significant changes in these levels after 3 weeks of occlusion [53]. However, in this study, patients with greater than two meibomian gland plugs per eyelid or patents with meibomian orifice irregularity were excluded. Therefore, while these results may not be applicable to all dry eye patients, it is important to consider each individual patient when determining whether or not to place punctal plugs [54].

To date, various modifications have been made to the initial silicone punctal plug, which is reflected in the wide variety of available products. Complications of punctal plugs are numerous and include extrusion, migration, canaliculitis or dacryocystitis, pyogenic granuloma formation, or discomfort [52].

If punctal plugs are not an option due anatomic anomaly or frequent punctal plug extrusion, permanent occlusion can be considered as a long-term treatment option. If possible, a trial of punctal plugs should be used prior to permanent closure. Punctal closure can be obtained via cautery or ligation, both of which have been traditionally used in aqueous deficiency dry eye. In thermal cautery, eyelid anesthesia is achieved and then a high-temperature cautery pen is placed into the punctum to the distal canaliculus. Heat is applied until tissue destruction occurs [55]. Various surgical techniques have been described for punctal ligation; however, no comparative studies exist. The goal is to create a raw surface within the canaliculus and suture the walls together to induce scarring and permanent closure [56, 57]. Minimal literature exists regarding the potential use of these techniques in evaporative dry eye secondary to MGD.

Concurrent pathology such as lower eye lid ectropion, eyelid retraction, or floppy eyelid syndrome should be assessed for and addressed if they are contributing to dry eye symptoms. Surgical correction of eyelid malposition reduces ocular exposure, and optimizes tear flow across the ocular surface by allowing the eyelids to efficiently pump tears into the lacrimal system. The specifics of surgical treatment for ectropion, eyelid retraction, and floppy eyelid syndrome are beyond the scope of this discussion.

Conclusion

The procedural options for treating blepharitis described in the first part of this chapter are relatively new and provide a different route to tackling this chronic disease with no truly curative treatment. Table 7.1 outlines the various treatment options discussed throughout this chapter. Intra-ductal probing, vector thermal pulsation, IPL, and microblepharoexfoliation were not used for treatment of blepharitis until a few years ago. There is still much that is unknown about the long-term efficacy of these treatments, but they provide additional options for patients who have failed traditional topical and systemic therapy.

Surgical procedures for chalazia, trichiasis, and distichiasis are well established. A reasonable goal in many cases is to control blepharitis well enough for these disorders to not occur.

Table 7.1 Procedural treatment of blepharitis and complications of blepharitis

Blepharitis	Intraductal meibomian gland probing	
	Vectored thermal pulsation	LipiFlow
		MiBoThermoflo
		TearCare
	Intense pulsed light	
	Microblepharoexfoliation	
Chalazion	Incision and curettage	
	Steroid injection	
Trichiasis	Radiofrequency ablation	
	Electrolysis	
	Cryotherapy	
	Trephination	
	Lamellar split	
	Wedge resection	
Evaporative Dry Eye	Punctal plugs	
	Permanent punctal closure	Suture ligation
		Thermal cautery
	Eyelid malposition repair	Ectropion
		Eyelid retraction repair
		Floppy eyelid repair

Compliance with Ethical Requirements The authors of this chapter do not have any conflicts of interest to report. The writing of this chapter did not involve carrying out any studies with human participants or animals performed by any of the authors.

References

1. Maskin SL. Intraductal Meibomian gland probing relieves symptoms of obstructive meibomian gland dysfunction. Cornea. 2010;29:1145–52.
2. Maskin SL, Alluri S. Intraductal meibomian gland probing: background, patient selection, procedure, and perspectives. Clin Ophthalmol. 2019;13:1203–23.
3. Maskin SL, Alluri S. Expressible meibomian glands have occult fixed obstructions: findings from meibomian gland probing to restore Intraductal integrity. Cornea. 2019;38:8.
4. Wladis EJ. Intraductal Meibomian gland probing in the management of ocular Rosacea. Ophthal Plast Reconstr Surg. 2012;28:416–8.
5. Syed ZA, Sutula FC. Dynamic intraductal meibomian probing: a modified approach to the treatment of obstructive meibomian gland dysfunction. Ophthal Plast Reconstr Surg. 2017;33:307–9.
6. Nakayama N, Kawashima M, Kaido M, Arita R, Tsubota K. Analysis of meibum before and after intraductal meibomian gland probing in eyes with obstructive meibomian gland dysfunction. Cornea. 2015;34:1206–8.
7. Sik Sarman Z, Cucen B, Yuksel N, Cengiz A, Caglar Y. Effectiveness of intraductal meibomian gland probing for obstructive meibomian gland dysfunction. Cornea. 2016;35:721–4.
8. Ma X. Lu Y. efficacy of intraductal meibomian gland probing on tear function in patients with obstructive meibomian gland dysfunction. Cornea. 2016;35:725–30.
9. Lane SS, DuBiner HB, Epstein RJ, Ernest PH, Greiner JV, Hardten DR, et al. A new system, the LipiFlow, for the treatment of meibomian gland dysfunction. Cornea. 2012;31:396–404.
10. Godin MR, Gupta PK, Kim T. The "eyelid facial": a review of meiboman gland heat treatments LipiFlow, MiBo Thermoflo, and intense pulsed light. In: Dry eye dis Pract guide. Thorofare: Slack Incorporated; 2019. p. 209–16.
11. Schiffman RM. Reliability and validity of the ocular surface disease index. Arch Ophthalmol. 2000;118:615.
12. Greiner JV. Long-term (12-month) improvement in meibomian gland function and reduced dry eye symptoms with a single thermal pulsation treatment: thermal pulsation treatment of dry eye. Clin Exp Ophthalmol. 2013;41:524–30.
13. Greiner JV. A single LipiFlow ® thermal pulsation system treatment improves meibomian gland function and reduces dry eye symptoms for 9 months. Curr Eye Res. 2012;37:272–8.
14. Hagen K, Bedi R, Blackie C, Christenson-Akagi KJ. Comparison of a single-dose vectored thermal pulsation procedure with a 3-month course of daily oral doxycycline for moderate-to-severe meibomian gland dysfunction. Clin Ophthalmol. 2018;12:161–8.

15. Kenrick CJ, Alloo SS. The limitation of applying heat to the external lid surface: a case of recalcitrant meibomian gland dysfunction. Case Rep Ophthalmol. 2017;8:7–12.

16. Badawi D. A novel system, TearCare® , for the treatment of the signs and symptoms of dry eye disease. Clin Ophthalmol. 2018;12:683–94.

17. Badawi D. TearCare® system extension study: evaluation of the safety, effectiveness, and durability through 12 months of a second TearCare® treatment on subjects with dry eye disease. Clin Ophthalmol. 2019;13:189–98.

18. O'Neil EC, Henderson M, Massaro-Giordano M, Bunya VY. Advances in dry eye disease treatment. Curr Opin Ophthalmol. 2019;30:166–78.

19. Toyos R, McGill W, Briscoe D. Intense pulsed light treatment for dry eye disease due to meibomian gland dysfunction; a 3-year retrospective study. Photomed Laser Surg. 2015;33:41–6.

20. Craig JP, Chen Y-H, Turnbull PRK. Prospective trial of intense pulsed light for the treatment of meibomian gland dysfunction. Investig Opthalmol Vis Sci. 2015;56:1965.

21. Liu R, Rong B, Tu P, Tang Y, Song W, Toyos R, et al. Analysis of cytokine levels in tears and clinical correlations after intense pulsed light treating meibomian gland dysfunction. Am J Ophthalmol. 2017;183:81–90.

22. Connor CG, Choat C, Narayanan S, Kyser K, Rosenberg B, Mulder D. Clinical effectiveness of lid debridement with BlephEx treatment. Invest Ophthalmol Vis Sci. 2015;56:4440.

23. Connor CG, Narayanan S, Miller W. Reduction in inflammatory marker matrix metalloproteinase-9 following lid debridement with BlephEx. Invest Ophthalmol Vis Sci. 2017;58:498.

24. Murphy O, O'Dwyer V, Lloyd-McKernan A. The efficacy of tea tree face wash, 1, 2-Octanediol and microblepharoexfoliation in treating Demodex folliculorum blepharitis. Cont Lens Anterior Eye. 2018;41:77–82.

25. Perry H, Serniuk R. Conservative treatment of chalazia. Ophthalmology. 1980;87:218–21.

26. Bensimon G, Huang L, Nakra T, Schwarcz R, Mccann J, Goldberg R. Intralesional triamcinolone acetonide injection for primary and recurrent chalazia: is it really effective? Ophthalmology. 2005;112:913–7.

27. Pizzarello L, Jakobiec F, Hofeldt A, Podolsky M, Silvers D. Intralesional corticosteroid therapy of chalazia. Am J Ophthalmol. 1978;85:818–21.

28. Watson A, Austin D. Treatment of chalazions with injection of a steroid suspension. Br J Ophthalmol. 1984;68:833–5.

29. Thomas E, Laborde R. Retinal and choroidal vascular occlusion following intralesional corticosteroid injection of a Chalazion. Ophthalmology. 1986;93:405–7.

30. Aycinena ARP, Achiron A, Paul M, Burgansky-Eliash Z. Incision and curettage versus steroid injection for the treatment of chalazia: a meta-analysis. Ophthal Plast Reconstr Surg. 2016;32:220–4.

31. Park J, Chang M. Eyelid fat atrophy and depigmentation after an intralesional injection of triamcinolone acetonide to treat chalazion. J Craniofac Surg. 2017;28:e198–9.

32. Shiramizu KM, Kreiger AE, McCannel CA. Severe visual loss caused by ocular perforation during chalazion removal. Am J Ophthalmol. 2004;137:204–5.

33. Hosal BM, Zilelioglu G. Ocular complication of Intralesional corticosteroid injection of a Chalazion. Eur J Ophthalmol. 2003;13:798–9.

34. Yagci AP, Egrilmez S, Sahbazov C, Ozbek S. Anterior segment ischemia and retinochoroidal vascular occlusion after intralesional steroid injection. Ophthal Plast Reconstr Surg. 2008;24:55–7.

35. Papalkar D, Francis IC. Injections for chalazia? Ophthalmology. 2006;113:355–6. author reply 356-357

36. Ben Simon GJ, Rosen N, Rosner M, Spierer A. Intralesional triamcinolone acetonide injection versus incision and curettage for primary chalazia: a prospective, randomized study. Am J Ophthalmol. 2011;151:714–718.e1.

37. Kezirian G. Treatment of localized trichiasis with radiosurgery. Ophthal Plast Reconstr Surg. 1933;9:260–6.

38. Ferreira IS, Bernardes TF, Bonfioli AA. Trichiasis. Semin Ophthalmol. 2010;25:66–71.

39. Sakarya Y, Sakarya R, Yildihm A. Electrolysis treatment of trichiasis by using ultra-fine needle. Eur J Ophthalmol. 2010;20:664–8.

40. Sullivan J, Beard C, Bullock J. Cryosurgery for the treatment of trichiasis. Am J Ophthalmol. 1976;82:117–21.

41. Majekodunmi S. Cryosurgery in treatment of trichiasis. Br J Ophthalmol. 1982;66:337–9.

42. Berry J. Recurrent trichiasis: treatment with laser photocoagulation. Ophthalmic Surg. 1979;10:36–8.

43. Bartley G, Lowry J. Argon laser treatment of trichiasis. Am J Ophthalmol. 1992;113:71–4.

44. Moore J, De Silva SR, O'Hare K, Humphry RC. Ruby laser for the treatment of trichiasis. Lasers Med Sci. 2009;24:137–9.

45. Pham RTH, Biesman BS, Silkiss RZ. Treatment of trichiasis using an 810-nm diode laser: an efficacy study. Ophthal Plast Reconstr Surg. 2006;22:445–7.

46. McCracken MS, Kikkawa DO, Vasani SN. Treatment of trichiasis and distichiasis by eyelash trephination. Ophthal Plast Reconstr Surg. 2006;22:349–51.

47. Ferraz LC, Meneghim RL, Galindo-Ferreiro A, Wanzeler AC, Saruwatari MM, Satto LH, et al. Outcomes of two surgical techniques for major trichiasis treatment. Orbit. 2018;37:36–40.

48. Moosavi AH, Mollan SP, Berry-Brincat A, Abbott J, Sutton GA, Murray A. Simple surgery for severe trichiasis. Ophthal Plast Reconstr Surg. 2007;23:296–7.

49. Chi MJ, Park MS, Nam DH, Moon HS, Baek SH. Eyelid splitting with follicular extirpation using a monopolar cautery for the treatment of trichiasis and distichiasis. Graefes Arch Clin Exp Ophthalmol. 2007;245:637–40.

50. Foulks GN, Bron AJ. Meibomian gland dysfunction: a clinical scheme for description, diagnosis, classification, and grading. Ocul Surf. 2003;1:107–26.

51. Lemp MA, Nichols KK. Blepharitis in the United States 2009: a survey-based perspective on prevalence and treatment. Ocul Surf. 2009;7:S1–14.

52. Jehangir N, Bever G, Mahmood SMJ, Moshirfar M. Comprehensive review of the literature on existing punctal plugs for the management of dry eye disease. J Ophthalmol. 2016;2016:1–22.

53. Tong L, Beuerman R, Simonyi S, Hollander DA, Stern ME. Effects of punctal occlusion on clinical signs and symptoms and on tear cytokine levels in patients with dry eye. Ocul Surf. 2016;14:233–41.

54. Song JS, Woo IH, Eom Y, Kim HM. Five misconceptions related to punctal plugs in dry eye management. Cornea. 2018;1:S58.

55. American Academy of Ophthalmology. Punctal occlusion for the dry eye. Ophthalmology. 1997;104:1521–4.

56. Murube J, Murube E. Treatment of dry eye by blocking the lacrimal canaliculi. Surv Ophthalmol. 1996;40:463–80.

57. Liu D. Surgical punctal occlusion: a prospective study. Br J Ophthalmol. 2002;86:1031–4.

Blepharitis: Future Directions

James J. Reidy

Introduction

Ophthalmologists have been struggling with the diagnosis and management of blepharitis for well over two centuries. While the common thread in all types of blepharitis is inflammation, the pathogenic mechanism(s) driving the inflammatory response remain poorly understood. Without a good understanding of the cause of blepharitis, physicians often end up treating only the effect(s) of the disease instead of the disease itself.

The Ocular Microbiome

During the last two centuries, anatomical and histological studies helped physicians to understand the basic structure and function of the eyelids. By the end of the nineteenth century, the germ theory of disease was fully established leading to rapid developments in the field of microbiology. Currently, identification of microbial species usually requires a culture-dependent analysis of the pathogenic organisms. However, these techniques are limited by both the culturability of certain microorganisms, as well as the time-consuming biochemical and phenotypic analyses that are required [1, 2]. More recently, culture-independent techniques have been employed to provide a more complete picture of the ocular microbiota [3]. Both 16S rRNA gene-based sequencing and matrix assisted laser desorption ionization-time of flight mass spectrometry (MALDI-TOF-MS) have enabled clinical microbiology laboratories to characterize a wide variety of bacteria, fungi, and viruses, as well as rapidly identifying those organisms utilizing standardized databases [2]. A significant percentage of the ocular microbiota is inhabited by bacterial species that have yet to be classified [3]. The role of these novel microbial species within the ocular microbiota remains to be elucidated.

The NIH Human Microbiome Project has helped to underscore the importance of the human microbiome in health and disease [4]. Metagenomic research has demonstrated a relationship between the gut microbiome and regulation of both innate and adaptive immunity [5]. Alteration of the human

J. J. Reidy (✉)
Department of Ophthalmology and Visual Science, The University of Chicago Medicine, Chicago, IL, USA
e-mail: jreidy@bsd.uchicago.edu

© Springer Nature Switzerland AG 2021
A. V. Farooq, J. J. Reidy (eds.), *Blepharitis*, Essentials in Ophthalmology,
https://doi.org/10.1007/978-3-030-65040-7_8

microbiome using treatment with specific probiotic strains has recently been shown to improve the clinical manifestations of autoimmune dry eye in an experimental model [6]. Future studies on the effect of the gut microbiome on ocular surface disease (OSD) and blepharitis may introduce novel treatment strategies to improve or prevent OSD.

Biomarkers for Disease

The diagnosis of blepharitis has been traditionally based on patient symptoms and clinical findings. Adjunctive diagnostic assessments help the clinician to refine the diagnosis and categorize the disease, select the most appropriate treatment, and evaluate the effects of treatment over time. Point-of-care testing for tear osmolarity, lactoferrin and tear IgE, and MMP 9 have been commercially available for several years. Many other proteins present in the tear film have been identified in the laboratory but are not yet commercially available. It would be most useful to have a test that is able to detect and quantify a panel of biomarkers that could identify dry eye, ocular surface inflammation, and meibomian gland dysfunction. Tear film protein assays suitable for clinical use include lactoferrin, MMP-9, MUC5AC, IL-6, IL-8, S100A8/9, and NGF [7]. Additional biomarkers are being identified with newer diagnostic modalities, and the clinical utility of these biomarkers will need to be explored further [8].

Omics and Bio-Data Science

In order to more fully understand the pathogenesis of blepharitis, examination of the underlying molecular mechanisms will help investigators diagnose disease, determine the prognosis, and design more effective treatments for the disease. Advances in sequencing, mass spectrometry, and bioinformatics have resulted in a rapid expansion in the understanding of the molecular mechanisms of human disease [9]. Omics is a relatively new field of study that characterizes and quantifies different types of biological molecules on a large scale. *Genomics* is the study of all of the genes that make up an organism, and how those genes interact with one another and the environment. Once the human genome was mapped, the function and structure of different genes could be studied and compared to other humans, as well as other species. Scientists soon realized that the genome is only partially responsible for the development of complex diseases. The localized environment that the organism is exposed to influences gene expression and metabolism that can ultimately trigger different disease states [9].

Both *proteomics*, the study of the structure and function of cellular proteins, and *metabolomics*, the study of low molecular weight compounds in a biological sample, can influence human health and disease [9]. Analysis of the proteomic profile of human tears has identified over 1500 proteins that could be potential biomarkers of ocular and systemic disease [8]. Jiang and co-authors [10] recently identified 48 metabolites that contributed to the incidence of dry eye using metabolomic analyses. Proteomic analysis in a group of patients with graft-versus-host disease (GVHD) following allogenic hematopoietic cell transplantation (AHCT) identified 13 proteins that may predict the development of the more severe forms of GVHD [11]. Tong el al [12] have noted a correlation between the severity of meibomian gland disease (MGD) and specific tear proteins (calgranulin A & B) in dry eye patients using proteomic analysis. These proteins may serve as useful biomarkers to detect and follow these disease processes, assist in the development of commercial test kits, and identify treatment strategies.

Increasingly, network and pathway-based analyses, *interactomics,* may be applied to ophthalmic diseases in order to gain further insights into disease-specific gene regulatory networks and cell signaling pathways [13]. These complex analyses are made possible by employing bio-data science methods, a synergistic marriage between the core disciplines of biology, computer science, as well as mathematics and statistics [14].

Senescence and Regenerative Medicine

Aging or senescence is a complex multifactorial process that affects the cellular components of the eye and adnexa, as well as the rest of the body. This process is driven by oxidative stress, damage to DNA and the repair process that follows, inflammation, metagenic signaling, telomere shortening, and immunosenescence [15].

Aging changes of the ocular surface include decreased goblet cell density in the conjunctiva, gradual telangiectasia of the eyelid margin, decreased IL-6 and IL-8 in the tear film, decreased tear film osmolarity, decreased tear volume, decreased tear film breakup time, and MG dropout [15]. The accumulation of advanced glycation end-products (AGEs) occurs in connective tissue leading to conjunctival chalasis, dermatochalasis, canthal laxity, loss of fibers from the orbicularis muscles, and intramuscular fibrosis [16]. The meibomian glands (MG) undergo acinar atrophy, thickening of cellular basement membranes, intraductal hyperkeratinization, shortening of the central ducts and ductiles, and lipogranulomatous inflammation resulting in decreased volume and quality of MG secretions [17]. Nien and colleagues [18] propose that altered PPARg (perioxisome proliferator-activated receptor gamma), a regulator of lipogenesis and sebocyte differentiation, may underlie the senescent changes observed in the MG.

There is a gradual decrease in immune function (immunosenescence), and conversely an overall increase in autoimmunity associated with aging [15]. The thymus gland undergoes an incremental involution leading to decreased T cells and decreased cytokine levels [15]. Persistent low-grade inflammation, such as occurs with ocular rosacea, may lead to tissue destruction associated with chronic macrocyte and lymphocyte activation. Elevations in IL-1, IL-6, IL-8, and TNFα have been observed [19].

Therapeutic strategies for age-related changes should be based on three principles: prevention of senescence, reversal of the pathologic processes involved in the aging process, as well as regeneration or replacement of the affected cells or tissue. The interdisciplinary field of regenerative medicine is focused on the repair, replacement, or regeneration of cells, tissues, or organs to restore impaired function resulting from any cause including aging, disease, congenital defects, or trauma [20]. In the future, the causes and effects of chronic blepharitis may, in part, be addressed using the varied methods employed in regenerative medicine that include the use of soluble molecules, stem cell transplantation, tissue engineering, genetic engineering, and advanced cellular therapy [21].

The use of hemoderivatives in the management of refractory dry eye disease, persistent epithelial defects, graft-versus-host disease, and neurotrophic keratitis have been widely adopted as adjunctive therapy of these disorders [22]. Both autologous serum (AS) and platelet-rich plasma (PRP) have been used successfully to treat number of different ocular surface diseases over the past 2-3 decades [23, 24]. These agents perform multiple functions similar to the normal tear film that include hydration and lubrication of the ocular surface, anti-inflammatory and antimicrobial properties, and enhancement of epithelial wound healing [22].

Stem cell therapy for the management of severe ocular surface disease has traditionally been reserved for severe acquired and congenital cornea limbal stem cell deficiency. In the past decade, there has been increasing interest in the use of mesenchymal stem cells (MSCs) to treat ocular disease [25]. These fibroblast-like cells are derived from the embryonic layer of the mesoderm and are self-renewing and able to differentiate into multiple, distinctive progenitor cells [26]. Although originally identified in the bone marrow, MSCs are also present in the umbilical cord, adipose tissue, and the corneal stroma [26]. Since they express neither major histocompatibility complex II (MHC-II), nor co-stimulatory molecules, they may be used allogeneically [27]. MSCs may be administered either intravenously [26], directly injected into or adjacent to the target tissue [22], or given topically [28]. The primary mechanisms of action of MSCs are as follows: *immunomodulatory* (decrease pro-inflammatory cytokines, increase anti-inflammatory cytokines, increase regulatory T cells, and modulate the balance of Th1 and Th2 cell populations) [22, 29]; *inhibition of angiogenesis* (decrease VEGF and MMP-2, and increases Thrombospondin1) [30]; *regenerative* (increase acinar cells within meibomian glands, increase conjunctival goblet cells, increase tear volume, improve tear film stability, and enhance corneal epithelial healing) [22, 28]; *cellular replacement* (differentiation to corneal epithelial cells and keratocytes, and glandular epithelium within the meibomian glands and possibly in the lacrimal glands) [28, 31].

As noted above, the rapid advances that are currently taking place in biology, computer science, laboratory science, and bio-data science across the globe will continue to advance our understanding of the pathophysiology of this disease and will improve our ability to diagnose and treat patients. Technology and hard work will reduce the time between discovery and development of a cure for a multitude of ocular diseases.

Compliance with Ethical Requirements

Conflict of Interest
James J. Reidy, M.D., declares that he has no conflict(s) of interest.

Informed Consent
No human studies were carried out by the authors for this chapter.

Animal Studies
No animal studies were carried out by the authors for this chapter.

References

1. Lee SE, Oh DH, Jung JY, Kim JC, Jeon CO. Comparative ocular microbial communities in humans with and without Blepharitis. Invest Ophthalmol Vis Sci. 2012;53(9):5585–93. https://doi.org/10.1167/iovs.12-9922.
2. Croxatto A, Prod'hom G, Greub G. Applications of MALDI-TOF mass spectrometry in clinical diagnostic microbiology. FEMS Microbiol Rev. 2012;36:380–407. https://doi.org/10.1111/j.1574-6976.2011.00298.x.
3. Dong Q, Brulc JM, Iovieno A, Bates B, Garoutte A, Miller D, et al. Diversity of bacteria at healthy human conjunctiva. Invest Ophthalmol Vis Sci. 2011;52(8):5408–13. https://doi.org/10.1167/iovs.10-6939.
4. Peterson J, Garges S, Giovanni M, McInnes P, Wang L, Schloss JA, et al. The NIH human microbiome project. Genome Res. 2009;19:2317–23. http://www.genome.org/cgi/doi/10.1101/gr.096651.109
5. Honda K, Littman DR. The microbiota in adaptive immune homeostasis and disease. Nature. 2016;535:75–84. https://doi.org/10.1038/nature18848.
6. Choi SH, Oh JW, Ryu JS, Kim HM, Im SH, Kim KP, Kim MK. IRT5 probiotics changes immune modulatory protein expression in the extraorbital lacrimal glands of an autoimmune dry eye mouse model. Invest Ophthalmol Vis Sci. 2020;61(3):42. https://doi.org/10.1167/iovs.61.3.42.
7. D'Souza S, Tong L. Practical issues concerning tear protein assays in dry eye. Eye Vis (Lond). 2014;1:6. https://doi.org/10.1186/s40662-014-0006-y.
8. Ahmad MT, Zhang P, Dufresne C, Ferrucci L, Semba RD. The human eye proteome project: updates on an emerging proteome. Proteomics. 2018;18(5-6):e1700394. https://doi.org/10.1002/pmic.201700394.
9. Lauwen S, de Jong EK, Lefeber DJ, den Hollander AI. Omics biomarkers in ophthalmology. Invest Ophthalmol Vis Sci. 2017;58(6):BIO88–98. https://doi.org/10.1167/iovs.17-21809.
10. Jiang Y, Yang C, Zheng Y, Liu Y, Chen Y. A set of global Metabolomic biomarker candidates to predict the risk of dry eye disease. Front Cell Dev Biol. 2020;8:344. https://doi.org/10.3389/fcell.2020.00344.

11. O'Leary OE, Schoetzau A, Amruthalingham L, Geber-Hollbach N, Plattner K, Jenoe P, et al. Tear proteomic predictive biomarker model for ocular graft versus host disease classification. Transl Vis Sci Technol. 2020;9(9):3. https://doi.org/10.1167/tvst.9.9.3.

12. Tong L, Zhou L, Beuerman RW, Zhao SZ, Li XR. Association of tear proteins with Meibomian gland disease and dry eye symptoms. Br J Ophthalmol. 2011;95:848–52. https://doi.org/10.1036/bjo.2010.185256.

13. Hu ZZ, Huang H, Wu CH, Jung M, Dritschilo A, Riegel AT, Wellstein A. Omics-based molecular target and biomarker identification. Methods Mol Biol. 2011;719:547–71. https://doi.org/10.1007/978-1-61779-027-0_26.

14. Goh WWB, Wong L. The birth of bio-data science: trends, expectations, and applications. Genomics Proteomics Bioinformatics. 2020;18:5–15. https://doi.org/10.1016/j.gpb.2020.01.002.

15. de Souza RG, de Paiva CS, Alves MR. Age-related autoimmune changes in lacrimal glands. Immune Netw. 2019;19(1):e3. https://doi.org/10.4110/in.2019.19.e3.

16. Feher J, Olah Z. Age-related changes of the eyelid. In: Cavallotti CAP, Cerulli L, editors. Age-related changes of the human eye. Aging in medicine: Humana Press. https://doi.org/10.1007/978-1-59745-507-7_2.

17. Obata H. Anatomy and histopathology of human Meibomian gland. Cornea. 2002;21(Suppl 2):S70–4. https://doi.org/10.1097/01.ICO.0000031084.62888.1E.

18. Nien CJ, Paugh JR, Massei S, Wahlert AJ, Kao WW, Jester JV. Age-related changes in the meibomian gland. Exp Eye Res. 2009;89:1021–7. https://doi.org/10.1016/j.exer.2009.08.013.

19. Mariani E, Pulsatelli L, Neri S, Dolzani P, Meneghetti A, Silvestri T, et al. RANTES and MIP-1α production by T lymphocytes, monocytes and NK cells from nonagenarian subjects. Exp Gerontol. 2002;37:219–26.

20. Greenwood HL, Singer PA, Downey GP, Martin DK, Thornsteinsdóttir H, Daar S. Regenerative medicine and the developing world. PLoS Med. 2006;3(9):e381. https://doi.org/10.1371/journal.pmed.0030381.

21. Dieckmann C, Renner R, Milkova L, Simon JC. Regenerative medicine in dermatology: biomaterials, tissue engineering, stem cells, gene transfer and beyond. Exp Dermatol. 2010;19:697–706. https://doi.org/10.1111/j.1600_0625.2010.01087.x.

22. Villatoro AJ, Fernández V, Claros S, Alcoholado C, Cifuentes M, Merayo-Lloves J, et al. Regenerative therapies in dry eye disease: from growth factors to cell therapy. Int J Mol Sci. 2017;18:2264. https://doi.org/10.3390/ijms18112264.

23. Jones L, Downie LE, Korb D, Benetez-del-Castillo JM, Dana R, Deng SX, et al. TFOS DEWS II management and therapy report. Ocul Surf. 2017;15:575–628. https://doi.org/10.1016/j.jtos.2017.05.006.

24. Merayo-Lloves J, Sanchez-Avilla RM, Riestra AC, Anitua E, Begoña L, Orive G, Fernandez-Vega L. Safety and efficacy of autologous plasma rich in growth factors eye drops for the treatment of evaporative dry eye. Ophthalmic Res. 2016;56:68–73. https://doi.org/10.1159/000444496.

25. Joe AW, Gregory-Evans K. Mesenchymal stem cells and potential applications in treating ocular disease. Cur Eye Res. 2010;35(11):941–52. https://doi.org/10.3109/0271368.2010.516466.

26. Zhang L, Coulson-Thomas VJ, Ferreira TG, Kao WW. Mesenchymal stem cells for treating ocular surface diseases. BMC Ophthalmol. 2015;15(Suppl 1):155. https://doi.org/10.1186/s12886-015-0138-4.

27. Ankrum JA, Ong JF, Karp JM. Mesenchymal stem cells: immune evasive, not immune privileged. Nat Biotechol. 2014;32(3):252–60. https://doi.org/10.1038/nbt.2816.

28. Beyazyildiz E, Pinarli FA, Beyazyildiz O, Hekimoglu ER, Acar U, Demir MN, et al. Efficacy of topical mesenchymal stem cell therapy in the treatment of experimental dry eye syndrome model. Stem Cells Int. 2014;2014:250230. https://doi.org/10.1155/2014/250230.

29. Nakashima H. Membranous nephropathy is developed under Th2 environment in chronic graft-versus-host disease. Med Hypotheses. 2007;69:787–91. https://doi.org/10.1016/j.mehy.2007.02.015.

30. Oh JY, Kim MK, Shin MS, Lee HJ, Ko JH, Wee WR, Lee JH. The anti-inflammatory and anti-angiogenic role of mesenchymal stem cells in corneal wound healing following chemical injury. Stem Cells. 2008;26:1047–55. https://doi.org/10.1634/stemcells.2007-0737.

31. Liu H, Zhang J, Liu CY, Wang IJ, Sieber M, Chang J, Jester JV, Kao WWY. Cell therapy of congenital corneal diseases with umbilical mesenchymal stem cells: Lumican null mice. PLoS One. 2010;5(5):e10707. https://doi.org/10.1371/journal.pone.0010707.

Index

Printed in the United States
by Baker & Taylor Publisher Services